Inner Peace Outer Beauty

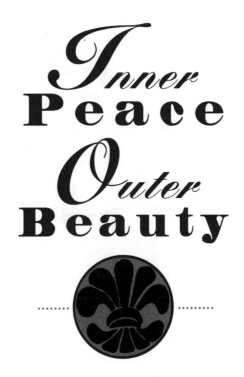

Inner Peace Outer Beauty

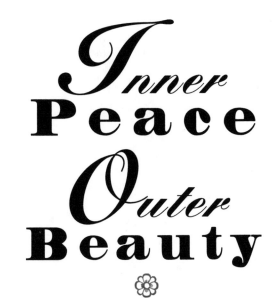

NATURAL

JAPANESE

HEALTH

and

BEAUTY

SECRETS

REVEALED

Michelle Dominique Leigh

ILLUSTRATED BY
Michelle Dominique Leigh

A CITADEL PRESS BOOK
Published by Carol Publishing Group

This book is presented as a collection of natural remedies and as an aid in understanding the theories and practices underlying their use. The book does not represent an endorsement or guarantee as to the efficacy of any remedy or of its preparation. The remedies are not intended to replace or supersede medical consultation and treatment.

Copyright © 1992, 1995 by Michelle Dominique Leigh

Originally published as *The Japanese Way of Beauty*

A Citadel Press Book
Published by Carol Publishing Group
Citadel Press is a registered trademark of
Carol Communications, Inc.

Editorial Offices
600 Madison Avenue
New York, NY 10022

Sales & Distribution Offices
120 Enterprise Avenue
Secaucus, NJ 07094

In Canada: Canadian Manda Group
One Atlantic Avenue, Suite 105,
Toronto, Ontario M6K 3E7

Manufactured in the United States of America
10 9 8 7 6 5 4 3 2 1

Carol Publishing Group books are available at special discounts for bulk purchases, for sales promotions, fund-raising, or educational purposes. Special editions can also be created to specifications. For details contact: Special Sales Department, Carol Publishing Group, 120 Enterprise Ave., Secaucus, NJ 07094

Library of Congress Cataloging-in-Publication Data

Leigh, Michelle Dominique
    Inner peace, outer beauty : natural Japanese health and beauty secrets revealed / by Michelle Dominique Leigh.
        p.   cm.
    "A Citadel Press Book."
    ISBN 0-8065-1628-3 (pbk.)
    1. Beauty, Personal.   2. Cosmetics—Japan.   3. Toilet preparations—Japan.   I. Title.
    RA778.L53 1995
    646.7'042'0952—dc20   94-43520
                                                                    CIP

CONTENTS

To wash one's hair, make one's toilet,
and put on scented robes;
even if not a soul sees one,
these preparations still produce an inner pleasure.

"Things That Make One's Heart Beat Faster"
Sei Shonagon, *The Pillow Book*, tenth century

INTRODUCTION

I began to gather the material for this book five years ago. The project originated in the most casual manner: I happened to notice, perched inscrutably upon a shelf at the local drugstore, a small paper envelope decorated with pink plum blossoms and birds, and the words *Nightingale Droppings* written in English. Feeling a bit like Alice down the rabbit hole, I couldn't resist buying the mysterious packet.

A Japanese friend translated the fine print: "Mix the droppings with warm water and massage into the face; you will get skin like a geisha's." Plus a considerate warning, "This product may reek somewhat." In the interest of broadening my cultural horizons, not to mention the alluring prospect of attaining geisha-like skin, I applied the faintly pungent, somewhat reeking, greenish substance to my face, massaged it in, let it sit there a few minutes for good measure, and rinsed it off. Something magical had happened—my skin seemed poreless, with a luster so silky, so polished that it felt brand new!

Undoubtedly, the Japanese beauty tradition offered more such esoteric delights, and I set out to discover them. I was surprised to find there were no books on the subject, either in English or Japanese. My friends, modern females in their twenties and thirties, professed complete ignorance in such matters, having put all their faith in the miracles of cosmetic science.

But occasionally I came upon a clue, some arcane-looking package with rustic calligraphy and paintings of gourds, vine leaves, or an ancient-looking landscape, and I would take it home, have it translated, and try it out. I learned that while many women of my generation knew nothing about their natural beauty tradition, their mothers and grandmothers did—and many still used the old techniques. These women passed their knowledge on to me just as they had received it: orally.

I documented what I learned, and continued my hunt for more, eventually sending questionnaires to women wherever I could find them, of all ages and in every part of Japan. The questionnaires came back with page after page of beauty advice, recipes, and wisdom. Though my original intent was to gather material of purely Japanese origin, I came to see that—as in any orally transmitted tradition that has evolved over centuries—there had been much borrowing from other cultures.

Realizing this, I relaxed my original parameters. I decided to focus on the techniques and concepts which had *become* Japanese, whatever their source. Further, I wished to focus on the living traditions and not on those which had become extinct—because in an empirically-based body of folk knowledge, those techniques which actually work are generally those that survive the centuries. As often as possible, I present the most recent versions of the old beauty techniques, for in general their modern adaptations have rendered them more harmonious with a twentieth-century lifestyle, and by the same token more accessible to the non-Japanese reader.

As I explored the Japanese beauty tradition I found that within it the realms of food, medicine, beauty, and even ancient religion and magic overlapped. The same foods that form a part of the everyday diet are those used in the healing and prevention of illness; they are also the ingredients used in beauty remedies. In this holistic system, the body and the mind are not separately considered; cures are often simultaneously external and internal, supplemented by mechanical methods like massage or pressure-point stimulation. The ingredients of the Asian herbal medicine tradition turn up in tonic teas, in the bath, in fragrant oils for the hair, as condiments for food, and in beauty treatments for the skin.

With the "green" movement growing stronger worldwide, the urge to return to nature for our medicines, foods, and beauty remedies has gathered momentum. Medical researchers and cosmetics scientists discover ever more astonishing properties in the botanicals used for centuries in folk traditions worldwide.

Along with plant-based external and internal beauty recipes, this book also includes explanations of the scrubbing massage, facial massage, scalp massage, and the Japanese approach to grace, serenity, and inner beauty.

Inner Peace, Outer Beauty is designed as a practical guide. It may be used as one would use a cookbook, dipping into it for a recipe as needed, or it may be used as a manual to devise a complete personal beauty regimen based on the extraordinary beautifying substances and methods of the Japanese tradition. Along with the opportunity to attain more beautiful skin, more luxuriant hair, and a lovelier body, *Inner Peace, Outer Beauty* may lead the reader to discover and cultivate the beauty within, to draw out and bring to life the soft elegance and subtle refinement that is nurtured by the Japanese approach.

How to Use This Book

The book is organized into three sections: face, hair, and body. In each section, the reader will find recipes and techniques which address every aspect of beauty care; basic regimens are also presented to serve as models for the reader who wishes to undertake a complete beauty routine.

The appendixes in the back of the book offer further information on tools and methods of preparation as well as a list of the ingredients included in the recipes, with suggestions about where they may be obtained. A list of mail-order sources for ingredients is provided as well.

PART ONE
THE BEAUTY OF THE FACE

INNER BEAUTY

As religions go, the Japanese Shinto-Buddhism combination is without doubt one of the most beautifying. Shinto teaches that the way to be is to have a well-polished heart; a bright-shining heart; a crystal-clear heart; a true heart; a straight-aiming heart. Buddhism promotes right-mindedness, calm, recognition of but detachment from negative thoughts and feelings, and compassion for others. In the midst of inclement emotional "weather," external difficulties, discomfort, and pressure, the Japanese Shinto-Buddhist maintains the focus of the inner eye, a softness and detachment that sometimes seems like imperviousness to the Westerner.

In the course of conducting research for this book, I talked with Japanese women and girls (and men and boys) of all ages about beauty. In answer to the question "What do you do to be beautiful?," more often than not the first response was not related to external care but to state of mind: "I look in the mirror for signs of negative feelings, like worry, jealousy, or anger, and if I see them I soften my face and my mind. I teach myself to hold bright, peaceful thoughts in focus and to turn away from unhappy, tense thoughts. I try to think about making other people happy. There cannot be external beauty if the mind and heart are not first carefully tended."

The beautiful woman has a serene face. She emanates a gentle brightness of spirit. This state of inner beauty is not always easy to achieve; sometimes it is a struggle; sometimes all that is possible is to present the appearance of that ideal inner beauty and peace. But magically, sometimes simply softening and brightening the face will lighten the heart as well.

The Japanese "bright, clear heart" is not to be confused with a state of mindless gaiety. Behind the smiling countenance of the Buddha is a deep awareness of suffering, which is the source of compassion. The eyes and smile are imbued with higher vision, fortitude, a kind of cool and detached all-accepting love. The woman who can emulate this demeanor may find that her inner being grows more beautiful in response, and that this state of serene inner beauty is a curiously simple matter of mental focus. For the Japanese, beauty starts from this essential depth: a delicate balance in a state of grace.

THE FACE WASH

*U*ntil the turn of the century, women in Japan were washing their faces with rice bran, azuki bean powder, and bush warbler droppings, just as they had done for a millennium. Even after Western-style soaps and cleansing creams were introduced, with their exotic cachet as fashionable luxury items, women would still follow up their cream or soap cleansing with a traditional powder scrub.

To the Japanese woman accustomed to the traditional face washes, soap seems overly harsh, while cleansing creams seem to lack the purifying and smooth-polishing properties of the bran, bean, and bird-dropping powders. The simple old-fashioned cleansers accomplished exactly what was needed: very thorough cleansing of the skin and gentle exfoliation of the surface, without stripping the complexion of its natural oils.

The traditional washes, which are not only cleansing but nourishing, healing, and lightening to the complexion, also lend themselves naturally to use in facial massage and treatment packs; unlike soap, any of the Japanese washes may be massaged into the skin and then left there for as long as one likes, providing beautifying benefits.

The purifying face-washing ritual is primary and central to the Japanese way of beauty. The effect of these washes is a complexion that gleams with a silky luster. This is the starting point for all other beauty treatments: skin that is fresh, pure, and renewed.

CHOOSING A FACE-WASHING TOOL

In determining the choice of washing bag, brush, sponge, or fingers for face-washing, consider skin type and immediate condition.

Drawstring Bags

In ancient Japan, ladies of the Imperial court washed their faces with silk, while commoners used cotton. The delicate fabric was fashioned into a tiny drawstring bag to be filled with washing powder—usually a combination of rice bran or azuki bean powder with camellia nuts—and the bag would be soaked in warm water in preparation for washing.

The washing bag or fabric mitt offers a good balance between gentleness and stimulation, and whether in cotton or silk, will be appropriate for most skin types.

Both silk and cotton bags are still produced commercially in Japan and made at home for face-washing. Much finer in texture than a Western-type washcloth, the bag of soft fabric performs a gentle sloughing of the face while the cleansing ingredients within nourish, polish, and purify the complexion. The bag's contents may be used for several consecutive washings, with the bag being carefully hung to dry between uses, and then the bag is emptied and washed and dried for repeated use. A woman who customarily uses the washing-bag technique will keep a small supply of bags on hand.

An alternative to the drawstring bag is simply to place a small pile of washing powder at the center of a gauze, muslin, or silk square, gather the ends together, and tie with a cord.

Face Brushes

The face brush is widely used in Japan for washing; this method supplies stimulation and efficient cleansing, with the soft and flexible bristles of the brush being very gently applied to the face in small rotating movements. While a facial brush or loofah will exfoliate the skin efficiently, these tools may be too stimulating for oily and sensitive skins, and certainly should be avoided by those with sunburned, blemished, or otherwise irritated skin.

Sponges

Soft sponges for the face include sea sponges and the delicate translucent sponge made from *konnyaku*, or devil's tongue root. The *konnyaku* sponge is said to encourage the elimination of toxins, imparting to the skin a dewy, jewel-like luster. Both the *konnyaku* sponge and the sea sponge are entirely nonabrasive, and are the implements of choice for sensitive, irritated skin or babies' skin.

Fingertips

Finally, the face may be washed with the fingertips, the simplest, most natural, nonabrasive, traditional method of all.

Whatever technique is chosen, the Japanese face-wash is both delicate and absolutely thorough. All movements should be soft and light and respectful of the skin—never hasty or rough—and at the same time diligent, aiming to purify every last pore. The Japanese mother will advise her daughter to wash her face as if she is polishing a rare treasure, a precious art object. Without doing damage to the fine surface, she must polish it to a gleam.

Steps in the Japanese face wash

- Apply oil to remove oil-soluble makeup and dirt. Massage gently. Wipe oil softly from face with cotton.
- Wash with water-moistened cleansing ingredient (using bag, brush, sponge, or fingertips) to remove remaining oil and water-soluble dirt. Water should be at body temperature.
- Rinse thoroughly with clear water, finishing with a few splashes of ice-cold water while patting the face vigorously all over.
- Using gauze, muslin, cheesecloth, or silk, gently pat the face dry.

17

Cleansing Oil

This first step in the face-cleansing process is designed to soften, loosen, and remove oil-soluble makeup and grime from the face. Almost any oil is suitable for this purpose, but the Japanese favorite is camellia oil.

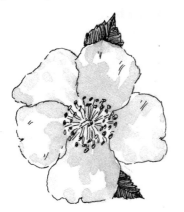

Actions:

Removes oil-soluble dirt and cosmetics

Indications:

All skin types
Use as often as needed prior to face-washing, especially at the end of the day

Ingredients:

Any pure natural oil:
camellia oil, sesame oil, safflower oil, shark's liver oil, walnut oil

Directions for Use:

Apply about a spoonful of oil to the face, rubbing gently with the fingertips.

Wipe the oil delicately from the face with cotton or gauze.

Rice-Bran Wash

Actions:

Cleanses	Softens	Lightens	Nourishes
Moisturizes	Smooths	Heals	

Indications:

All skin types
Recommended for use instead of soap on babies'
  skin, blemished skin, and sensitive skin
Daily use

Ingredients:

Fresh pure rice bran, powdered

Directions for Use:

Fill a small silk or cotton drawstring bag very tightly with rice bran, ground to the texture of fine powder.

The bag is soaked in a bath or basin for a few minutes, then gently squeezed. The milky liquid which seeps through the cloth is evidence that the bag is ready to use.

With a gentle massage motion, rub the bran bag over the face, then rinse. Alternative method: mix rice bran with warm water in the palm of the hand, then massage onto the face; rinse.

The rice-bran bag may be used for 2 to 3 washings, once moistened. Between uses, hang it up in a dry place. After several washings, the bag must be emptied, washed carefully with soap, and dried prior to further use.

NOTE: To keep rice bran fresh, store carefully sealed in a cool, dry location.

Sometime in the dim reaches of ancient history, the Japanese discovered that the rich bran of the rice grain had some extraordinary properties. Used for washing natural wood floors, rice-bran water not only removed dirt but supplied subtle oils, and the effect over time was to give the wood a deep and lustrous gleam. Women who used the water left over from washing white rice to wash dishes or to add to the bath (the Japanese have a traditional penchant for recycling their resources) noticed that their skin seemed to grow ever more beautiful: moist, smooth, soft, and fine. Hair washed and rinsed in the rice-bran water was well-cleansed, but lost none of its natural sheen, because the rice bran nourished the tresses with just the right amount of oil. Many of the very oldest women in Japan grew up using nothing but rice bran for washing their faces and bodies, and it is to rice bran that they give the credit for their remarkable supple, smooth-textured complexions.

Pink Bean Powder

The pink of azuki bean powder! A pale and perfect pink: the pink of cherry blossoms, the pink of sweet rice cakes, the pink of the rice eaten to celebrate Girls' Day.

Pink bean powder has been used as a face wash in Japan for 1,200 years, and it is still popular today. Court beauties of ancient Japan would scrub face and body with small silk bags containing azuki powder; modern Japanese women use cotton bags or apply the creamy powder directly to the skin. The azuki bean is valued in Japan for its medicinal properties and its lacquer-red hue; its effectiveness as a beauty treatment is truly time-honored. The delicate wash, with its fine particles of bean, sloughs and deep-cleans the skin, leaving it glowing, tightened, and silky-smooth.

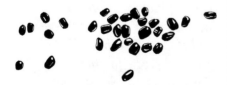

Actions:

Cleanses
Exfoliates
Lightens
Softens
Stimulates

Indications:

All skin types
Daily use

Ingredients:

Azuki beans

Preparation:

Azuki beans must be briefly roasted to remove moisture. Using a heavy skillet, roast on the stovetop over medium high heat for 5 to 10 minutes, stirring constantly. (If beans lose their red color, they have been roasted too long.)

Grind the beans into a very fine powder, using a coffee or grain mill (traditionally, the beans were stone-ground). Sift. The powder should be as fine and soft as face powder.

Store in a sealed jar; keep free of moisture.

Directions for Use:

Mix bean powder with a little warm water in the palm of the hand. Rub the bean-cream over the face and massage softly before rinsing.

Pearl Barley and Pink Bean Powder

Actions:

Cleanses
Clears
Exfoliates
Lightens
Softens
Stimulates
Detoxifies
Purifies

Indications:

All skin types
Recommended for troubled skin, skin marked by
    freckles, warts, and age spots
Daily use

Ingredients:

Pearl barley (*Coix Lacrymae Jobi*)
Pink powder of azuki beans

Preparation:

Place pearl barley seeds in a skillet to dry-roast
over medium high heat for 5 to 10 minutes,
stirring constantly.

Grind the seeds into a fine powder using a grain
or coffee mill. Sift.

Store in a sealed jar kept free of moisture.

Directions for Use:

In the palm of the hand or in a face-washing
bag, add the two ingredients in equal amounts,
moisten with warm water, and massage gently
over the face. Rinse.

Pearl barley, also known as Job's tears, is medicinal, the traditional Japanese skin-healer, spot, freckle and wart-remover, complexion-lightener, and general beautifier. One who is troubled by imperfect skin is advised to get plenty of sleep and undertake a pearl barley cure. Eating pearl barley porridge, drinking pearl barley tea, and applying pearl barley to the face is the ancient Oriental holistic remedy.

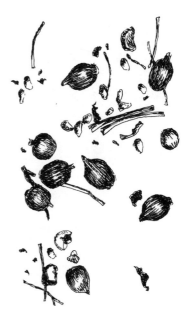

Crushed Camellia Nuts

The camellia nut, the kernel from the fruit of the winter-blooming camellia tree, has supplied Japanese women for centuries with treasured camellia oil, used for beautiful skin and tresses. The camellia flower itself is a symbol of feminine beauty, the vivid red or warm pink of its blooms glowing in gentle grace against the cold white of winter snow.

Actions:

Cleanses
Exfoliates
Moisturizes

Indications:

Not recommended for oily or sensitive skin
Recommended for dry and normal skin
Weekly use

Ingredients:

Nuts from the camellia tree, *Camellia linne Japonicus*
Rice bran

Preparations:

Gather camellia fruits just after they appear on the tree in autumn or winter; extract the nuts inside, dry, and store.

Directions for Use:

Place some camellia nuts in a face-washing bag along with some rice bran. Strike the bag several times against a hard surface, causing gentle crushing of the nuts and the emergence of the oil.

Moisten the bag in warm water until a milky liquid emerges, then rub gently over the face to cleanse.

Rinse.

Golden Honey Wash

Actions:

Cleanses
Nourishes
Soothes
Softens
Purifies

Indications:

All skin types
Recommended for aging, dry, sensitive,
  blemished, and babies' skin
Daily use

Ingredients:

Natural honey
Rice bran or bean powder

Directions for Use:

In the palm of the hand, mix washing powder
with a little honey and warm water, massage
gently and thoroughly into the skin, then rinse.

Another method: after soaking a *nukabukuro*
containing washing powder, dribble some honey
onto the bag before washing the face with it.
Rinse.

Pure golden sweetness and light, the honey of summer bees is a natural treasure for beauty. Appreciated in all parts of the world for its curative and nourishing properties, honey has long been important in Oriental herbal medicine.

In Japan, honey soap is available in liquid and solid forms, and is particularly valued for its delicate soothing benefits—lovely for calming irritated sensitive skin. The rice bran and honey mixture will help babies' diaper rash and teenagers' troubled skin. A treat for aging or dry skin, honey helps to replenish and "hold in" moisture while gently stimulating the circulation and supplying nutrients, giving the skin softness and a luminous, honeyed glow.

23

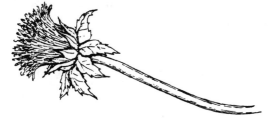

Black Sugar Wash

Black sugar, or kurozato in Japanese, is not really black, but a deep golden-brown. This most primitive of sugars is all powdery, crumbly chunks and pebbles, like some magically sweet earth-mineral. It is, in fact, very rich in minerals and vitamins which nicely nourish the skin. This sugar has the dark taste and aroma of molasses, and molasses may be substituted if the true black sugar can't be had. In Japan, a traditional soap is also made from kurozato—the young appreciate this black sugar substance for its ability to calm acne and overactive oil glands, and women of a certain age credit black sugar with revitalizing and smoothing the tired or dull complexion.

Actions:

Cleanses
Nourishes
Moisturizes
Revives
Smooths

Indications:

All skin types
Recommended for oily or troubled skin
Daily use

Ingredients:

For Black Sugar Syrup:
   9 ounces (250 cc) dark unrefined sugar
   2 cups (480 ml) pure spring water
For Wash:
   Black sugar syrup
   Rice bran, bean powder, or bush warbler
      droppings

Preparation:

To make syrup, heat the sugar and water in a nonmetal pan over a gentle flame. Stir constantly, removing scum from the surface of the mixture as it appears.

When the mixture thickens, remove from heat and allow to cool. Transfer the liquid to a glass bottle and store in the refrigerator.

Directions for Use:

Follow directions for Golden Honey Wash, page 23.

Bush Warbler Droppings

Actions:

Cleanses
Lightens
Nourishes
Tones
Smooths
Moisturizes
Exfoliates

Indications:

Not recommended for sensitive or allergy-prone skin
Beneficial for aging skin, oily, blemished, or rough skin
Use once or twice weekly

Ingredients:

Dried bush warbler droppings

Preparation:

If you keep a bush warbler or two to supply you with *uguisu no fun*, the birds' diet should be high in protein, fat, and greens. Recommended are salt-free freshwater fish powder, soybean powder, pulverized green leaves, and furry caterpillars.

The droppings are collected, spread in the sun to dry completely, ground to a fine powder with a mortar and pestle, then transferred to an airtight container for storage. (Moist droppings will irritate the skin and should not be used.)

In February in Japan, when days are still dark and bitter with cold, when snow still flutters occasionally through the air, amid this wintry landscape suddenly appears the warm pink of the blossoming plum tree, the first whisper of spring. To join the plum blossoms in the early welcome, the bush warbler moves from her winter home in the tall bamboo to her spring residence in the plum tree. Snow, blossoms of girlish pink, small birds singing of spring: these images are easily linked with the vision of the delicate white skin and faintly pink-tinged cheeks of the geisha.

But a bit of humor relieves the too-sweet enchantment—it is the bird's droppings that give the geisha her pearly pallor. This esoteric beauty wash is viewed by modern young women as an embarrassing eccentricity, but someone is still using it, for packets of dried bush warbler droppings are available even in my corner drugstore. Beauties of old would make a daily stop at the local bird store for their own personal supply. While the idea of massaging bird droppings onto the face may at first seem strange, the greenish-white stuff is effective; the face is left looking satiny, poreless, and brand new!

Directions for Use:

Mix the powder with a little warm water to moisten, then apply to the face, massaging gently.

Uguisu no fun may be left on the face for up to 20 minutes as a pack, in which case its smoothing, lightening, and exfoliating benefits will be intensified.

Uguisu no fun may be mixed with rice bran for another effective face wash. (Unlike rice bran, bush warbler droppings, once moistened, should not be saved for subsequent use.)

NOTE: This unusual treatment is included as it is one of the most respected of the Japanese beauty secrets.

Seaweed Scrub

Actions:

Cleanses
Stimulates
Detoxifies
Revives
Tones

Indications:

All skin types
Recommended for aging skin
Daily use

Ingredients:

Any dried edible sea plant without additives, in leaf or powder form.

Preparation:

Soften dried seaweed by soaking in tepid water for 20 minutes. (Powdered seaweed may be used as is.)

Directions for Use:

Place softened seaweed in a washing bag—powdered seaweed may be used in the same manner—moisten in warm water, and gently massage the face. Rinse.

Japan is a land of the sea, with fishes and sea plants and tiny marine creatures of infinite variety forming an important part of the daily diet. The Japanese seaweed bath is like a miniature ocean, adrift with swirling salty green, a poetic metaphor like the tiny twisted bonsai pine in a Japanese garden. Scrubbing the face and body with vivid green, red, or brown sea plants is a practice that is not only aesthetically pleasing, but also extraordinarily nourishing to beauty and health. Seaweed is as tonic to the skin as a dip in the ocean, swimming amid the fishes and the sea flowers. Aging skin will appreciate the seaweed scrub for its powers of refreshment and invigoration.

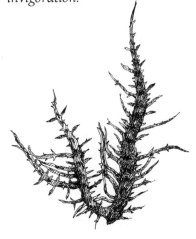

Cold Water Splash

The cold-water face splash, practiced after thoroughly cleansing the face, is a pure and simple method for stimulating circulation, activating cell metabolism, and giving a healthy glow to the complexion. About fifteen splashes of ice-cold water, morning and night, will keep wrinkles at bay, say Japanese grandmothers. After soaking for a long time in a hot bath, turn on the cold-water faucet and let the water rush onto your face. If you pat your face briskly at the same time, you increase the benefits. When not in the bath, fill a basin with icy water, then splash the face with both hands.

This practice reminds me of the Japanese fondness for sitting under cold waterfalls in the chill of winter—a discipline derived from Zen Buddhism's "training to harden oneself." The at-home version is not nearly so rigorous.

FACIAL WATERS

Perhaps because the Japanese archipelago is a naturally wet place, with seas and oceans, abundant freshwater lakes and rivers, and a moist climate generous in rainfall and mists, the traditional Japanese way of beauty utilizes only the lightest of plant waters and tonics to gently preserve the skin's natural moisture. While in the Western natural beauty tradition there is much that is rich, oily, and creamy, the Japanese way favors the limpid, translucent, and pure.

The Japanese woman considers the application of facial water, rinse, or tonic lotion to be an essential part of the daily beauty ritual. As simple and subtle as these waters may seem, they perform an important function: the protection of the complexion against sunlight, weather, and dehydration. Many of the waters act to further purify the skin, lighten freckles and age spots, heal blemishes, and stimulate circulation as well. Because almost all of the transparent or translucent facial waters help the skin to retain moisture, they are used faithfully by older women to delay the appearance of wrinkles, lines, dry skin, and other signs of aging.

There are facial waters and lotions appropriate to each season: cucumber for summer, black sugar or rice for winter, plum for spring, loofah vine for autumn. Loofah vine water has long been the most beloved of the facial water genre; it was originally used by women rice-farmers to protect their skin from sun damage and drying winter winds.

Each recipe presented here offers its own unique array of treatment benefits to the skin—some emphasize purification, others softening and smoothing, and

---

When and how to apply waters, rinses, and tonics

- For waters and tonics, after cleansing the face and patting it dry, apply water or tonic to a cotton pad or a small folded piece of gauze; pat gently onto the face. Air dry.
- If using a rinse, prepare the rinse in a basin with tepid to cool water. Splash the rinse repeatedly onto the cleansed face, catching the overflow in the basin. Air dry after patting gently with gauze or cotton.

---

still others nourishment and protection. With daily use, over time, the complexion will respond by becoming healthier and more beautiful. Because the waters contain only light natural plant oils and nutrients, there is no clogging of the pores; the skin receives treatment while continuing to breathe.

A Note on Preservation

When preparing any of the facial waters or tonics, you can add a natural preservative to make them last a little longer. This is especially useful if you are going to follow a treatment plan for an extended period of time. A few drops of tincture of benzoin (in proportions of 1½ teaspoons (7 ml) benzoin per 1 cup (240 ml) of liquid, or ¼ ounce benzoin per 8 ounces liquid) will prolong the life of the solution. (Benzoin is astringent, antiseptic, soothing, and mildly stimulating.) After adding benzoin, place the mixture in a clean, well-sealed glass bottle and store in the refrigerator. Prepare the waters and tonics in small batches, and shake well before each use. Any changes in the appearance or odor of the facial water are signs that it is no longer fresh.

Water of Lotus Root

Actions:

Tones
Heals
Calms irritations

Indications:

All skin types
Recommended for blemished or sensitive skin
Daily use or as needed

Ingredients:

2 tablespoon (30 cc) fresh lotus root
1¼ cups (300 ml) pure spring water

Preparation:

Chop lotus root into small pieces, then soak in cold water in a nonmetal pot for one day.

Simmer the mixture over a gentle fire until the water is reduced by half. Filter through gauze, discard the solids, and allow to cool.

Store in a glass bottle in the refrigerator for no more than 3 days.

Directions for Use:

Apply with cotton or gauze to a cleansed face. If the skin is very irritated or blemished, do not apply moisturizer or foundation, but gently pat on some loose powder.

Lotus: nelumbo nucifera, is a member of the Nymphaeaceae *family. Not only the name but the entire plant is mystically beautiful, with its lily pad leaves and its lush meditative blossoms, and its segmented root that reveals a cutout flower pattern when sliced, like something by Matisse.*

Lotus root is an ancient part of the Japanese diet, and a traditional healing plant as well. The recipe given here may also be used to soothe rashes and prickly heat.

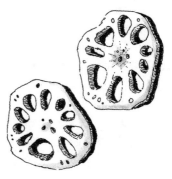

Honorable Spirits of Rice

Women who work in Japan's "water trade"—the term given to the nighttime entertainment business, which revolves largely around drinking—are said to apply clients' leftover sake to their skin to keep it beautiful.

Sake is a fermented beverage—not really a wine—made from rice. It was originally created by the Japanese gods and it is still employed in Shinto wedding rites and as a ritual offering to the spirits of the ancestors. The best sake comes from the same parts of Japan that produce the most beautiful women; these are the areas of crystal-pure fresh water and the highest-quality rice.

The sake divinity is a jealous goddess who is thought to react badly to the presence of human women in breweries, but in early Japan it was the most beautiful young virgins who were called upon to do the rice-chewing and spitting that was the old-fashioned way to begin the fermentation process. The sake thus made was known as "beauty" sake.

Sake is said to lighten age spots and cool and soothe irritated or sunburned skin.

Actions:

Smooths
Lightens
Calms
Cools

Indications:

All skin types
Daily use

Ingredients:

Sake (Japanese rice wine)

Directions for Use:

Simply apply plain *sake* to the skin with fingers, cotton, or gauze. Do not rinse.

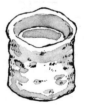

First Water of Rice

Actions:

Nourishes
Moisturizes
Heals
Smooths
Softens

Indications:

All skin types
Recommended for dry skin
Daily use

Ingredients:

Pure rice bran powder
Water

Preparation:

Add a few spoonfuls of finely powdered rice bran to a basin of cool water.

Directions for Use:

Splash the rice bran water repeatedly over a freshly cleansed face.

This water may be rinsed with a final, cool, plain-water splash, but some prefer not to rinse the bran water off, leaving it to lightly moisturize the skin.

Before cooking polished white rice, it is ritualistically washed, usually for about five minutes, until the originally milky-looking washing water looks quite clear. The first water is the water containing the highest quantity of fine particles of bran from the polishing process.

In the old days, when rice-polishing was accomplished without the use of abrasive polishing compounds, the first washing water contained only bran and was safely nourishing to the skin.

These days, unless you know your polished rice is free of such additives, it is best to approximate the first water of rice by mixing it yourself.

Cucumber Juice Tonic

Cucumber tonic is one of the two classic beauty waters in the Japanese tradition. Cucumber tonic is used in the morning; its season is summer. Loofah vine water is for nighttime and winter is its season.

The cucumber's potency in beauty-making is extraordinary and diverse, as it is useful against wrinkles, lines, freckles, blemishes, sunburn, dry skin, oily skin, roughness, and almost any other problem one could name.

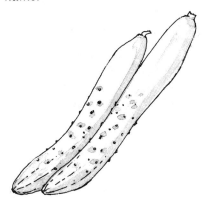

Actions:

Cleanses
Cools
Heals
Softens lines
Moisturizes
Lightens
Soothes

Indications:

All skin types
Recommended for oily skin, sunburned skin, blemishes and wrinkles
Daily use

Ingredients:

5¼ ounces (150 cc) chopped fresh cucumber
2 cups (480 ml) *shochu* or vodka
(*Shochu* is a tasteless colorless distilled spirit containing 20 to 45 percent alcohol.)

Preparation:

Add cucumber to *shochu* in a wide-mouthed glass container and seal tightly. Store in a cool, dark location for one month, then remove the solids by straining through gauze.

Directions for Use:

After cleansing the face, apply cucumber juice tonic to the face by patting gently with a tonic-soaked gauze. Do not rinse.

(A little fresh cucumber juice direct from the vegetable may be used for tonic as well.)

NOTE: Some very sensitive skins may be irritated by cucumber, in which case it should not be used.

Ceremonial Green Tea Tonic

Actions:

Stimulates
Calms irritations
Soothes sunburn
Astringes
Tones
Lifts
Firms

Indications:

All skin types
Recommended for aging or tired skin, rough skin
Daily use

Ingredients:

2 teaspoons (10 cc) powdered green tea
½ cup (120 ml) pure spring water
Ceramic tea bowl
Small bamboo tea whisk

Preparation:

Warm the tea bowl in hot water. Rest the whisk (a small metal whisk may be substituted) in hot water. Empty and dry the tea bowl.

Place powdered tea in the bowl with hot water, and whip with the whisk until frothy.

Excess tea may be refrigerated and used for 2 to 3 days.

Directions for Use:

When tea has cooled to room temperature, apply to the face with cotton or gauze. Do not rinse.

Chilled tea is particularly refreshing in hot weather; add ice cubes or refrigerate.

This elegant and simple beauty recipe returns green tea to one of its ancient uses as an external curative. The venerable leaf-green beverage, referred to by fifth-century Chinese poets as "froth of the liquid jade," occupies the place of honor in the Zen tea ceremony, where it is prepared, tasted, and admired in an atmosphere of profound and timeless contemplation.

To properly enact the beauty ritual and participate in the relaxing aesthetic tradition of tea, the mind must be calm. Select your tea bowl with care—it should be a ceramic bowl of some grace and dignity—and give your focused attention to the details of preparation. Movements are slow, peaceful, and imbued with quiet awareness of the moment.

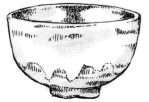

Loofah Vine Water

Plant your loofah seedling in April, when the young spring is well begun, the ground soft, the sunshine warm. You will watch the process of the plant as it forms leaves and buds, then yellow flowers, until finally, toward summer's end, the long green loofah gourds hang heavy from the vine.

On the night of the last full moon of September, cut the vine stem at a point between 50 and 70 centimeters from the ground, then place the living cut end inside a large 1.8 liter sterilized sake bottle. Wrap the opening to seal it from air and dust, then leave the bottle to fill. It may take anywhere from one night to several days for this to occur.

Loofah vine water is the most trusted of the traditional Japanese lotions. It is lightening, protective, moisturizing, and healing, and thus it has long been considered the ideal beauty water for the woman who wishes to protect her fair and delicate complexion from the harsh cold of the Japanese winter and the strong heat of the Japanese sun. Loofah vine water is also produced commercially by many Japanese companies.

Actions:

Protects
Lightens
Moisturizes
Heals
Softens

Indications:

All skin types
Recommended for aging skin, winter skin, sun-exposed skin, dry skin
Daily use

Ingredients:

Loofah vine sap
(Optional: Japanese *sake* or *shochu* (vodka))

Preparation:

Once you have collected the fresh loofah vine sap, you can proceed with one of two methods to preserve and store it.

The vine-water purists advise adding nothing to the sap, just to filter it through gauze and transfer it to small sterilized glass bottles, to be stored in the cold and dark (refrigerator).

Another method, more commonly advised, is to add either *sake* or *shochu* (1 part alcohol to 5 parts sap) and proceed as above, with small bottles to be refrigerated.

Directions for Use:

Apply to a freshly cleansed face by patting gently with cotton or gauze. Do not rinse.

Water of Pine

Actions:

Stimulates
Soothes
Purifies
Protects

Indications:

All skin types
Recommended for aging skin
Daily use

Ingredients:

A big handful of pine needles
1¼ cups (300 ml) pure spring water

Preparation:

Add pine needles to the cold water and allow to infuse for several hours. Then bring to a boil, immediately lower the fire, and simmer for 5 minutes.

Filter the liquid through gauze and discard the solids.

Cool before use; refrigerate. Store in the refrigerator in a glass bottle for no more than 3 days.

Directions for Use:

Apply to a freshly-cleansed face with cotton or gauze. Do not rinse.

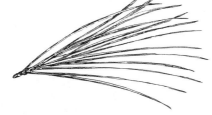

Pine, in Japan, is all that is fresh, new, and auspicious. Purity, long life, and good luck. The tree of the New Year, when all is renewed and begins again.

When the gardener attends to the old pine tree in our garden, he not only prunes it with artistry, creating ever more graceful twists and elegant curves, he lovingly trims the needles, bunch by bunch, longer here, shorter there, thinning and shaping until each tiny detail of the tree is aesthetically perfect, and the overall composition is one of breathtaking harmony, the soul of the tree made visible. The process takes two ten-hour days, and at the end of it the old man stands back from his work, gives a quiet grunt of approval, bows, and takes his long bamboo ladder and goes off to other pine trees in other gardens.

Pine water is advised for older skin, which is thought to benefit from its properties of renewal, stimulation of the circulation, and moisture protection. Pine is also tonic, antibacterial, and slightly astringent, so it imparts to the complexion a superb sensation of clean refreshment.

Tonic of Fresh Fruit Peel

Karube-san, who was the midwife for the birth of my daughter, is a down-to-earth country woman in her seventies. She has delivered thousands of babies, and she is a font of wisdom regarding tonic teas, health-giving herbs, and strengthening foods. Seeing her expansive knowledge of folk medicine, I asked her about beauty. Her response: eat a lot of fish, black beans, and burdock—beauty comes with health—don't worry about things, and rub fruit peels on your face after eating the fruit. She claims to have used the fruit peel treatment all her life, and her skin is indeed fine.

Actions:

Tones
Nourishes
Refreshes

Indications:

All skin types
Daily use

Ingredients:

Any fresh fruit peel or rind

Directions for Use:

Rub the fruit side of the peel gently over a cleansed face. Pat dry with gauze; do not rinse.

Dry skin will appreciate peach or apricot peel; normal skin will like grape; lemon peel and grapefruit will do nicely for oily skin; sensitive skin will benefit from pear. For blemishes, use apple.

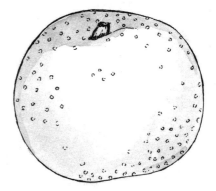

Pink Plum Sake

Actions:

Exfoliates
Smooths
Purifies

Indications:

All skin types
Daily use

Ingredients:

7 or 8 *umeboshi* (pickled plums)
1 cup (240 ml) *sake* (rice wine)

Preparation:

To extract the salt from *umeboshi*, place them in a jar of warm water. Change the water several times daily over a period of two days.

Put the saltless *umeboshi* with the *sake* in a glass jar or bottle and seal. When a week or ten days have passed, filter the liquid through gauze. Discard the solids.

Transfer to small bottles if desired.

Directions for Use:

Apply with cotton or gauze to a cleansed face. Do not rinse.

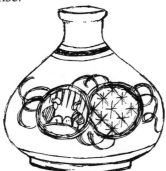

Japanese women have long considered sake to be beneficial to the skin when applied directly or used in the bath. To combine the skin-silkening rice wine with the talismanic umeboshi—which is thought to cure most anything, and bring luck besides—was an inspired idea.

Many of the most legendary natural Japanese beauty secrets were originated by geisha. The pink plum sake was found to eliminate the geisha's corns within days. From this experiment it was deduced that the same lotion applied to the face would smooth and exfoliate, resulting in the fresh delicacy that characterizes the ideal complexion. This too proved delightfully effective, and the geisha told their friends the sushi chefs about it. The sushi chefs applied pink plum sake to their hands, rough and reddened from the daylong washing and slicing of cold fish. The sushi chefs told their wives, and the wives told their friends, and so on, until pink plum sake was a secret known to everybody, even to me, who was told by the little old lady who sells vegetables down the street.

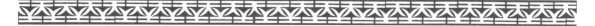

Black Sugar Rinse

Black sugar rinse is a simple, sweet treatment for skin that suffers from stress or fatigue.

Actions:

Revives
Nourishes
Stimulates
Moisturizes
Lightens
Heals blemishes and rashes

Indications:

All skin types
Recommended for dry skin, tired skin, winter-
    dry or chapped skin, aging skin, troubled skin
Daily use

Ingredients:

Pure unrefined sugar; molasses may substitute
Pure spring water

Preparation:

Dissolve some dark sugar or molasses in tepid water.

Directions for Use:

Splash sugar water repeatedly onto a freshly cleansed face. Do not rinse.

OILS AND EMOLLIENTS

*I*n the days when Japanese women coated their faces in heavy layers of opaque white powder, the skin was first prepared by the application of oil, pomade, or oil-and-wax cerate as a makeup base. This makeup base served two purposes—it facilitated the even application and long-lasting adherence of the powder, and it acted as a protective barrier between the drying powder and the skin. Thus, the role of the makeup base was to sit on the surface of the skin rather than to penetrate it, acting as a kind of protective glue.

Oils have traditionally been used to lubricate the skin during facial massage, as solvents in cleansing the face of makeup, and as remedies for specific skin problems. Traditional hair oils or pomades were also frequently used on the skin; these were composed of waxes, resin, nut oils, and fragrant essential oils—cassia, bergamot, citrus, geranium, clove, and sandalwood—and ingredients such as plum kernel oil or rose water. Beauty-oil makers concocted secret blends of essential oils and mixed them with carrier oils like sesame or walnut. Such oils,

---

When and how to apply oils and emollients

- For massage, apply plain oil or oil mixed with water to the freshly cleansed face, proceed with massage, and finish by wiping softly with gauze or cotton. A water, rinse, or tonic lotion may be applied if desired.
- As a makeup base, mix only a few drops of oil—camellia oil is best for this purpose—with water, then apply to the face with the fingertips.
- As a night treatment, apply plain oil or oil mixed with water to the cleansed face, massaging lightly with the fingertips.
- To remove makeup, apply oil to the face with the fingertips, rubbing and massaging gently, then wiping carefully with cotton or gauze. Proceed with water-cleansing.
- To keep eyelashes and eyebrows lustrous, a tiny amount of camellia or sesame oil may be applied nightly, after removing makeup. It is said that this practice encourages luxuriant growth. Camellia oil may be applied as a daytime eyebrow dressing; just a single drop on an eyebrow comb will tame the unkempt brow.

---

though originally created for use on the hair, gradually became popular for the skin, and were reputed to be medicinal and beautifying, healing blemishes, softening skin, and acting as tonics to the complexion.

With the disappearance of the white-powdered face and the stiff, elaborately-dressed hairstyles of earlier eras, the oils and emollients used in natural beauty care have themselves become simpler and lighter. Today, oils without added fragrance or waxes are used primarily to soften, smooth, and lubricate. Still, the same traditional oils are favored—camellia oil being the oil of preference, followed by sesame, safflower, walnut, and shark's liver oils. Complexions which require no additional oil benefit from the oil-free lubrication offered by aloe vera gel.

THE JAPANESE FACE MASSAGE

Massage is so much a part of Japanese life that it is taken for granted. Massage—a casual everyday version of the formal pressure-point shiatsu—is incorporated into dance and exercise classes, sports-team workouts, and is a standard service at the beauty salon, where the shampooist delivers a brief but exquisitely effective massage to forehead, scalp, neck, and shoulders. Children massage their parents; friends massage friends. I have watched entire classes of kindergarten children take turns at giving their teacher's shoulders an energetic pummeling.

When very young, the Japanese girl is taught that facial massage is an important part of the daily beauty ritual, just like washing. This simple practice is thought to be the most important of antiaging treatments; women of all ages massage their faces in order to delay the appearance of wrinkles and lines, and to soften them when they are already present. By delicately exercising and stimulating the muscles and tissue of the face, circulation and cell metabolism are activated, with the visible result of a fresher, more vital-looking complexion.

With regular facial massage, deadened, tired areas seem to brighten; tight, tense areas seem to soften and relax; expression lines are smoothed; sags, shadows, and droops are diminished. The features seem softer, more youthful, plumped up with life. The skin texture grows silky. Dirt trapped in the pores is coaxed to the surface, and the pores seem to breathe.

Massage carried out correctly on a daily basis will gradually restore elasticity and tone to the skin. The manual relaxation of habitually tensed muscles of the face (for example, the mouth and eye areas) will enable one to begin to recognize and eliminate the facial signs of worry, anxiety, anger, and stress, all of which contribute to an older-looking appearance with their pinched-inward or downward-pulling effects.

Based as it is on the ancient art of shiatsu, the finger-pressure massage which stimulates the *tsubo,* points on the body which correspond to specific internal organs and which are said to help release profound energies and enable the body to function in a smoother, more balanced and efficient way, the Japanese face massage is believed to benefit the entire being, not just the face.

The face massage is practiced nightly, after a thorough cleansing of the face. Because most benefits are gained when the pores are relaxed and open, first steam the face briefly over a basin of hot water or by holding the face close to a steaming towel. Doing the massage while soaking in the bath is pleasant and effective. The eyes should be closed for maximum relaxation.

To avoid damage to the skin caused by tugging or pulling, an emollient must be applied to the face. Choose from Japanese camellia oil, sesame oil, walnut oil, safflower oil or shark's liver oil. For oily or blemished skins, aloe gel may be used instead of oil, if desired. Oil that is warmed slightly before application is delightful.

Because the massage will help any nourishing ingredients to penetrate the skin, one of the liquid skin-foods like black sugar extract, molasses, or honey can be applied to the face before adding the oil. About a tablespoon of oil should be used—enough so that the fingers glide smoothly over the skin's surface. The massage is not designed to exfoliate; no abrasive powders or grains should be used.

The massage is usually practiced with the fingertips held together, pressing firmly with the fingerpads of forefinger, middle finger, and sometimes ring finger as well. To determine the proper technique, which may be described as delicate but penetrating, imagine that your skin is very fine silk, thin and easily stretched or torn. When moving across an area of the face, skin should not be displaced. The basic movements in the Japanese face massage are extremely gentle circular gliding strokes, straight strokes, and simple static pressure. The latter technique is effected by pressing firmly and rather deeply with the fingertips, with the pressure sustained for about five seconds each time. As strong a pressure as is comfortable may be applied.

When finished massaging, remove oil by gently wiping with cotton or gauze moistened with a tonic lotion. An oily skin should be cleansed of oil by washing and then toned.

43

The basic facial massage consists of the following strokes and movements:

Forehead:

A. Using the four fingers of each hand, spread fingers at eyebrow level so that little fingers touch at the lower center of forehead, and forefingers meet the hairline at the temples. Move fingertips up the forehead in straight strokes, applying pressure on the upward movement only. Do ten repetitions.

B. Using the forefinger and middle fingers of both hands, place forefingers with tips touching, middle fingers with tips touching, at the center of the forehead, and stroke outward, pulling from center forehead to hairline, using pressure only on the outward movement. Do ten repetitions.

C. Using the forefinger and middle fingers of both hands—the two fingers pressed against one another firmly—place the right-hand fingers at the inner end of the right eyebrow, the left-hand fingers at the left eyebrow. Spiraling in small circular glides, stroke up and out from the middle, ending at the hairline in the upper area of the forehead. Do ten repetitions.

Nose:

A. Using any two fingers pressed together, stroke downward from the bridge of the nose to the tip, using pressure only on the downward stroke. Do fifteen repetitions.

B. Using two pressed-together fingers of each hand, stroke straight up on either side of the nose. Use pressure only on the upward stroke. Do ten repetitions.

Eyes:

A. Using the pressed-together middle and ring fingers of each hand, stroke along the upper eyesocket, moving softly from the inner to outer edges. The same is done for the lower eyesocket. This stroke uses almost no pressure; it is designed to relax and release tension. Do ten repetitions each.

B. Apply static pressure to the upper eyesocket with the four fingers of each hand, arranged so that the little fingers press at the inner edges, forefingers at the outer. The same is done for the lower eyesocket. Do five repetitions each.

Mouth:

A. Using the pressed-together forefinger and middle finger of each hand, stroke outward above the lip, starting just below the nose and moving horizontally to the point where the smile crease occurs. The same movement is carried out below the lips, on the upper part of the chin. As always, use pressure only on the outward movement. Do ten repetitions.

Chin and Cheeks:

A. Using the pressed-together forefinger and middle finger of each hand, stroke outward from the center of the chin up to the lower cheek area, pressing only on the upward stroke. Do ten repetitions.

B. Using the same two fingers, move from the lower, inner cheek area toward the outer edge of the face, next conducting the same upward and outward movement from the edge of the mouth, and finally, from the nostrils. Use pressure only on the upward stroke. Do ten repetitions each.

C. Using the separate forefinger and middle finger of each hand, place hands so that the forefingers are next to the nose on the upper cheekbone edge, and the middle fingers are by the nostrils. Stroke straight out, moving toward the outer edge of the face. Use pressure only on the outward stroke. Do five repetitions.

D. Using the same spiraling glide movement described in Forehead, C, stroke from the center of the chin to the upper jawline and from the edge of the mouth to the upper outer cheekbone edge, pressing only on the upward strokes. Do ten repetitions each.

E. Apply static finger pressure to the cheek area by spreading the four fingers of each hand so that the little fingers are at the level of the mouth, in the smile-crease spot, with the forefingers just above the top outer cheekbone edge, and the other fingers spread evenly between the two end-points. Do five repetitions.

Neck:

A. Using the pressed-together forefinger and middle finger of each hand, stroke downward along the length of the neck. Do ten repetitions.

B. Using the spiraling stroke, move directly downward on the neck, just on either side of the Adam's apple. Do ten repetitions.

TREATMENTS, PACKS, AND RUBS

The face pack is a relatively recent Japanese beauty tradition. The oldest women in Japan today remember using egg whites or cucumber juice in this fashion, but not much else. In the Japanese tradition, the most important nourishment for the skin comes internally, from proper diet. When women did apply treatment substances to their faces for short periods of time, they generally used liquids: plant juice, sugar water, oil, or egg.

As minimal and subtle as these simple packs may seem, they are nonetheless effective. Applied with or without a rice-paper face-pack mask, the liquid pack is still a popular Japanese beauty treatment.

The less ephemeral Western-style face pack, with its thicker, creamlike texture and its various combinations of active ingredients, has inspired new uses for the traditional Japanese beauty-care substances. Rice bran, black sugar, pearl barley powder, soybean flour, and the various fruits, vegetables, flowers, and green leaves make effective, enchanting pack mixtures.

(Although purely Western pack ingredients are also used by Japanese women, sometimes alone and sometimes in combination with the Japanese substances, I do not include these familiar ingredients here.)

Many of the treatments are applied in a manner similar to the facial waters—that is, they are left on the skin without being rinsed, and in some cases reapplied frequently during the course of the day. Other treatments are applied only to the problem area as "spot packs," then rinsed. These treatments provide remedies for specific skin problems, and as such are designed to be used as cures, and discontinued when the skin condition improves.

The "rubs" described here offer a more active version of the face pack, a potent treatment version of the facial massage. The rubs, like the packs, are meant to be rinsed.

As an occasional boost to circulation and stimulant to cell activity, and as a now-and-then dose of concentrated nourishment and treatment for specific conditions, the pack is the perfect remedy. Packs are generally used once a week or so, but depending on the type of pack and one's particular skin type and needs, as often as two or three times a week might be desirable. If you are seeking to lighten the complexion, revive tired skin, or clear up blemishes, the appropriate treatment or pack must be applied with regularity over a prolonged period of time. Very stimulating or drying packs should be used no more than once a week, for excessive use can lead to irritation or an overly oily or dry condition.

When and how to apply treatments, packs, and rubs

- Before any of the following applications, the face is thoroughly cleansed and steamed briefly over a basin of hot water or by sitting in a hot bath. Pat dry.

Pack:

- If using a liquid pack, soak a gauze or rice-paper mask in the pack liquid as described previously and apply to the face. If the pack is the creamy spreadable type, apply an even layer over the face, avoiding the eye area and lips. (Camellia oil or black sugar water may be applied to these areas to nourish and smooth.) The pack may be applied to the neck area if desired. Allow the pack to remain on the skin for the recommended period, usually between five and thirty minutes. Lie down and relax, or soak in the bath, remembering that a too-hot bath will be likely to interfere with some packs by making them melt and drip off. To remove the pack, apply warm water and rub gently with the fingertips. Once the pack is entirely removed, finish with a cold-water splash. Pat gently dry.

Treatment:

- Pat gently onto the cleansed face with fingers, cotton, or gauze. Leave to dry; do not rinse. (Reapply during the day as needed.) Some treatments are applied as "spot packs," in which case the method is as for packs, but application is limited to the affected area.

Rub:

- Massage gently onto the cleansed face for five to ten minutes. Follow with a thorough rinsing and pat dry.

Pink Bean Powder Pack

Any of the Japanese beans may be used in a pack for nourishment, deep cleansing, and smoothing of the skin.

Actions:

Cleanses   Nourishes
Lightens   Heals
Smooths

Indications:

All skin types
Weekly use

Ingredients:

Azuki bean powder
Honey

Preparation:

Mix the two ingredients into a smooth cream.

Directions for Use:

Apply to a freshly cleansed face, and leave on for 20 minutes before rinsing.

Three-Powder Pack

Actions:

Stimulates
Soothes
Tones
Nourishes
Astringes
Cleanses

Indications:

All skin types (but buckwheat sometimes causes an allergic reaction, in which case it should be eliminated)
Recommended for tired skin
Weekly use

Ingredients:

Buckwheat flour (*soba* flour)
Rice flour
Soybean flour (*kinako*)

Preparation:

Mix equal amounts of each flour with enough warm water to make a paste.

Directions for Use:

Apply the mixture to a freshly cleansed face, leave on for 20 minutes, then rinse.

Black sugar or honey may be added to the pack if desired.

Buckwheat, rice, and soybean are three standards of Japanese cuisine, each of which also offers nourishment when used as external skin-food.

49

Rice Bran Pack

With a supply of fresh rice bran on hand, one can enjoy a simple but complete rice-bran beauty regimen: rice bran for cleansing, rice bran water for toning and moisturizing, rice bran as a treatment pack. Rich in "skin vitamins" B and E along with nourishing minerals and rice germ oil, rice bran may also be eaten. (And don't forget rice bran for bathing, washing dishes, and polishing wood floors. . . .)

Actions:

Moisturizes
Nourishes
Smooths
Stimulates
Heals irritated skin
Combats free radicals

Indications:

All skin types
Recommended for troubled skin
Use once or twice a week

Ingredients:

Rice bran
Rice flour

Preparation:

Using about 30 percent rice flour, mix with rice bran, then add warm water to make a creamy paste.

Directions for Use:

Apply the pack thickly to a freshly cleansed face, then leave it to work for 15 minutes. Rinse.

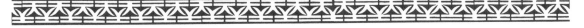

Pearl Barley Porridge Pack

Actions:

Purifies
Clears skin of imperfections

Indications:

All skin types
Recommended for skin that is troubled,
   blemished, or marked by freckles, warts, or
   age spots
Use as frequently as desired

Ingredients:

Pearl barley
Pure spring water

Preparation:

Using a blender or a grain or coffee mill, grind
pearl barley to a fine powder.

Simmer the powder with an equal amount of
water in a nonmetal pot, stirring constantly for
5 to 10 minutes.

Allow to cool at room temperature.

Directions for Use:

Apply the pearl barley porridge to a freshly
cleansed face. Leave the pack on for 15 to 20
minutes, then rinse thoroughly.

Pearl barley is the very first thing that comes to mind when there is any kind of skin trouble. Pearl barley has the virtue of being both powerfully medicinal and utterly mild and unstimulating. The pearl barley treatment is long-term and combines the internal and the external, with pearl barley taken daily, and pearl barley applied to the skin in whatever form is preferred: wash, pack, or tea-lotion.

51

Sesame Pack

When my son was three he went to a Japanese Montessori school, and one of his favorite activities there was grinding sesame seeds with a child-size mortar and pestle. Goma o suru is the name for sesame-grinding; the same expression is used to mean overflattering someone. Keep grinding sesame seeds long enough and you get sesame butter, a nice image for the process of buttering someone up.

Actions:

Nourishes
Moisturizes
Heals
Soothes

Indications:

Not recommended for blemished skin
Recommended for dry skin, sunburned skin, windburned skin
Use weekly or as needed

Ingredients:

Sesame seeds

Preparation:

Using a mortar and pestle, grind sesame seeds until they are completely pulverized into a paste-like sesame butter.

Directions for Use:

Apply a layer of sesame butter to the face (as always, freshly cleansed) and allow it to remain for 20 minutes. Rinse thoroughly.

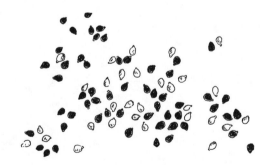

Simple Tofu Pack

Actions:

Nourishes
Softens
Smooths
Calms

Indications:

All skin types
Recommended for sensitive or tired skin
Use as often as desired

Ingredients:

Fresh tofu
Rice flour

Preparation:

To drain some of the liquid from tofu, place an appropriate amount in a piece of gauze and squeeze, discarding the liquid.

Mix tofu with enough rice flour to make a creamy paste.

Directions for Use:

Apply the tofu-flour mixture to a cleansed face; allow it to remain for 15 to 20 minutes, then rinse.

Japan is a land of paradox. It intrigues me that a country famous for its silence and serenity is really a rather noisy place. And some of my favorites among everyday Japanese sounds are those that echo from the traditional past: songs of the sellers of tofu, watermelons, hot steamed sweet potatoes, and bamboo poles.

These days the whistles, tunes, and peddlers' sing-song chants waft in endless repetition from tapes played on the roving trucks' loudspeakers, but the sounds are the same as the old sounds. "Tofu, tofu, delicious tofu . . . housewives, how about it? Tofu, tofu, delicious tofu. . . ."

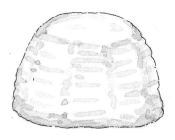

Winter Salad Face Pack

Japanese salads are delicate and subtle creations, usually artful and surprising combinations of ingredients, each chosen for its appropriateness to season and occasion—by its color, form, and mood; its freshness; and its ability to harmonize with its fellow ingredients.

Bits of black hijiki seaweed, sweet slices of baby tangerine, aromatic slivered pink-pickled ginger, raw grated daikon radish, and red perilla leaf are some of the refreshing surprises I've encountered in Japanese salads. Always, ingredients are cut, sliced, grated, minced, or decoratively carved with perfect style. The Japanese "beauty salad" here may be improvised in the same way, choosing vegetables in season in a combination that strikes your fancy and harmonizes with your mood.

Actions:

Smooths
Softens
Nourishes
Stimulates metabolism of the skin

Indications:

All skin types
Recommended for rough or dry skin, winter skin
Weekly use

Ingredients:

Fresh vegetables in any combination: carrots, cabbage, cucumbers, tomatoes, celery, lettuce, daikon (Japanese radish), spinach, aloe, soybean, sprouts
Rice flour (optional)
Camellia oil (optional, recommended if skin is very dry)

Preparation:

Vegetables may be finely grated, then mashed using a mortar and pestle or a blender.

There are two variations of this salad pack: one makes use of the mashed vegetables as they are, the other uses juice obtained by squeezing the substance through gauze. If you choose the latter, squeeze to get juice.

Directions for Use:

For variation I, apply the vegetable mash to a cleansed face and cover with a gauze or rice-paper face-pack mask. Relax for 15 to 20 minutes, then rinse.

For variation II, add a little rice flour—and camellia oil if desired—to the freshly squeezed vegetable juice. Apply the mixture to a cleansed face and leave on for 15 to 20 minutes before rinsing.

The Rice-Paper Face-Pack Mask

The rice-paper face-pack mask is a gloriously simple invention. Designed to make it possible to apply liquid treatment packs to the face, it has cutout eyes and mouth and a slitted nose-flap. The rice paper's porosity enables it to absorb liquid readily, while its strength prevents tearing. Delicate, lightweight, and disposable, this natural material serves its purpose with elegant efficiency. Gauze is another material employed in making face-pack masks, but the very slight stiffness of paper endows the paper mask with superior ease of handling. See the appendix for the cutout diagram.

Japanese Honeysuckle Pack

The delicate white honeysuckle flower seems the perfect accompaniment to the long, slow, dreamy, bee-buzzing days of midsummer. The seeming fragility of the fragrant blossoms belies the vigorous strength of the plant, which is described in my gardening book as a kind of garden-devouring monster that has escaped from cultivation to invade the entire civilized world. Japanese honeysuckle has ancient medicinal uses in the Orient, being respected as a treatment for all kinds of illnesses, and the flowers are well known for their healing effect on damaged skin.

Actions:

Heals
Purifies
Astringes

Indications:

All skin types
Recommended for blemished or irritated skin
Use weekly or as needed

Ingredients:

1 tablespoon (15 cc) honeysuckle flowers or buds
1 cup (240 ml) pure spring water
Rice flour

Preparation:

Prepare an infusion of the flowers by boiling the water in a nonmetal pot, removing from heat, and adding the honeysuckle flowers to the water. Allow to infuse for 15 minutes.

Mix the flower tea with enough rice flour to form a creamy paste.

Directions for Use:

Apply to a freshly cleansed face, and leave on for 20 to 30 minutes before rinsing.

October Persimmon Pack

Actions:

Lightens
Nourishes
Soothes
Heals

Indications:

All skin types
Weekly use

Ingredients:

One ripe persimmon
Rice flour

Preparation:

Mash the persimmon, using a mortar and pestle, then strain through gauze to obtain juice.

Add enough rice flour to the persimmon juice to form a creamy paste.

Directions for Use:

Apply pack to a freshly cleansed face and allow to remain for 15 to 20 minutes. Rinse.

The Japanese persimmon tree has a poetic soul. During early winter, it seems that every persimmon tree in the land is adorned by a final single fruit of brilliant orange, alone in sun-colored splendor amid the bare black branches, set like a jewel against the backdrop of snow.

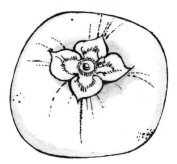

Summer Melon Pack

The melon is accorded a place of great honor in the Japanese food store. Waiting to be sold, it sits majestically upon the highest shelf (emperor of grapes and tangerines), protected by white latticed padding, a splendid globe of palest green, emerald, or veined eggshell-white. The Japanese have a fondness for round things: round fruits like plums and oranges, round white rice balls, the round full moon of October, the soft round cheeks of little girls. The melon, with its cool juicy sweetness, has a fresh purity that is aesthetically most Japanese: light-flavored, fragrant, crisp-textured, and beautiful to see, with the inside-outside surprise of playful color contrast.

Actions:

Soothes

Lightens

Tones

Indications:

All skin types

Recommended for skin irritations, sunburn, and to lighten freckles and age spots

Weekly use

Ingredients:

Any edible melon: watermelon, cantaloupe, honeydew, Persian

Preparation:

Mash ripe melon using a mortar and pestle.

Directions for Use:

Apply the mashed melon to a cleansed face, cover with a gauze or rice-paper face-pack mask, and leave on for 15 minutes before rinsing.

A quick and simple way to benefit from melon juice is to rub the rind's fruit side over the cleansed face, leave several minutes, then rinse.

58

Honey Lemon Camellia Pack

Actions:

Exfoliates
Softens

Indications:

All skin types
Recommended for rough or dull skin
Use as frequently as desired

Ingredients:

A spoonful of honey
A few drops of lemon juice
A few drops of camellia oil

Directions for Use:

Mix the three ingredients together and apply to a cleansed face. Let the pack remain for 15 minutes, then massage briefly before rinsing.

This combination of the sweet, the tart, and the flowery is like an elegant Japanese dessert, all liquid, translucent yellows, and golds.

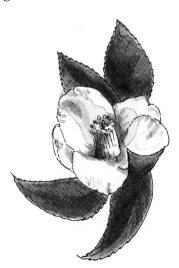

59

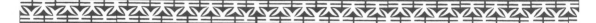

Black Sugar Honey Pack

Either of these sweet, mineral-rich substances makes a quick and effective beauty treatment. The skin circulation is stimulated while the complexion is nourished, soothed, and calmed.

A c t i o n s :

Cleanses
Nourishes
Moisturizes
Revives
Soothes

I n d i c a t i o n s :

All skin types
Recommended for tired or rough skin
Use as frequently as desired

I n g r e d i e n t s :

Black sugar syrup (for recipe see chapter on face
    washes)
or
Honey
    (A little rice flour may be added if a thicker
    consistency is preferred.)

D i r e c t i o n s   f o r   U s e :

Apply either sugar syrup or honey directly to the freshly cleansed face, massaging a little; leave on between 5 and 15 minutes. Rinse.

Whipped Egg-White Pack

Actions:

Tightens
Tones
Astringes

Indications:

Not recommended for dry skin
Recommended for oily or aging skin
Use as often as desired

Ingredients:

Egg white

Preparation:

Whip egg white into a stiff meringue.

Directions for Use:

Apply meringue to a freshly cleansed face, leave on for 15 to 20 minutes, then rinse.

(Unwhipped egg white may be used in the same way.)

There is a sake store near my house that is old—all shadows and dark wood, with centuries of dust in the corners. A tall, dignified old man inside sits behind his long wooden desk, adding up sums on his abacus and writing down the numbers. Along with the big and small bottles of sake, beer, and shochu, there is always a large basket of fresh chicken eggs for sale, and whenever I walk by the shop, the sight of these eggs, piled in a pleasing mound, creamy matte white with bits of straw here and there, draws my eye and fills me with an indescribable feeling of comfort.

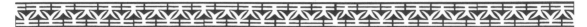

Salty Bancha Tea Eyelid Compress

One of the Japanese women I talked with while doing research for this book said to me, "I heal everything with tea." That tea—the Japanese and the western types come from the same bush—is medicinal is often forgotten, because the beverage is such a familiar everyday one. Tea has the dual virtue of being both stimulating and soothing, which makes it useful as a comforting, reviving drink when one is tired, or as an external remedy for fatigued eyes, which are effectively relaxed and refreshed by it.

Actions:

Cleanses
Stimulates
Soothes inflammation
Reduces puffiness
Astringes

Indications:

Recommended for tired or puffy eyes
Use as needed

Ingredients:

1 tablespoon (15 cc) *bancha* tea
1¼ cups (300 ml) pure spring water
1 pinch sea salt

Preparation:

Simmer tea leaves and water in a nonmetal pot for 20 minutes, then cool and filter 3 times through fine silk, discarding the solids.

Use only when freshly made.

Directions for Use:

Apply lukewarm tea to eyelids by soaking gauze folded into small squares to make compress pads. Lie down and relax with the tea compresses on the eyelids.

Aloe Eye Cooler

Actions:

Soothes
Cools
Relaxes

Indications:

Recommended for tired eyes
Use as needed

Ingredients:

Fresh aloe vera or *aloe arborescens* leaves

Preparation:

Slit a leaf lengthwise to expose the inner gel, then cut to the right size for the eyelid area.

Directions for Use:

Apply the leaf gel-side down to the closed eyelids while lying down for 15 minutes or so.

Many Japanese homes have a big potted aloe plant sitting conveniently outside the front door. The plant is known the world over as an effective soother of minor burns; in Japan the curative gel is also used to cool and relax the eyes.

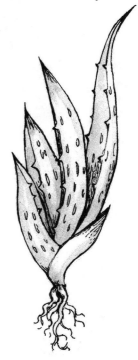

Sea-Green Seaweed Pack

Vivid green strips of soft wakame (seaweed) stick smooth and slick to the skin—an emerald marine masque to surprise skin cells into action.

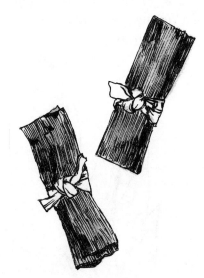

Actions:

Tones
Stimulates
Detoxifies
Refreshes
Combats sun damage
Cleanses

Indications:

All skin types
Recommended for tired skin, aging skin, sunburned skin, oily skin, dry skin
Use weekly or as desired

Ingredients:

Wakame seaweed (*Undaria pinnatifida*)

Preparation:

If *wakame* is fresh and unsalted, simply rinse.

If *wakame* is fresh and salted, soak in clear water for 15 minutes after rinsing.

If *wakame* is dried, soak in clear, cold water for 20 minutes, then rinse.

Directions for Use:

Apply strips of soft wet *wakame* to the cleansed face, leave on for 20 to 30 minutes, then remove and rinse.

SPOT TREATMENTS
(FOR PIMPLES AND BUMPS)

To hasten the departure of pimples by drawing out toxins, purifying, soothing, and encouraging drying and healing processes, the following remedies may be tried. In every case, apply directly to the area to be treated.

- Fresh **turnip** juice (obtained by grating the turnip and squeezing through gauze) mixed with sea salt may be dabbed onto blemishes several times a day. Don't rinse.
- **Chrysanthemum** leaves may be bruised with the fingers or a mortar and pestle, and the juice applied to pimples as often as desired, without rinsing.
- *Jinenjo*, or **mountain yam**, may be washed, grated raw, and applied as a spot pack (held in place with a wet piece of gauze if necessary, or mixed with rice flour to stiffen), left on for twenty minutes, then rinsed.
- A bit of fresh **garlic** juice can be applied (*only* to the blemish) or a charred garlic clove may be rubbed lightly against a troublesome spot. As always with garlic, sensitive skin should abstain.
- The leaves of **mugwort** may be bruised with the fingers or a mortar and pestle to obtain the juice, which is applied to the blemish several times daily, without rinsing. Another way to use mugwort is to apply the mashed leaves as a spot pack, covering the spot pack with a fresh mugwort leaf. Rinse after twenty minutes.
- **Persimmon** juice may be applied to a blemish several times daily; no rinsing is needed.
- The juice from grated **daikon (radish)** may be applied to blemishes several times a day, without rinsing.
- Fresh **aloe** gel may be applied often to blemishes to encourage scarless healing. No rinsing is needed.

BEAUTY TEAS
FOR FACE AND HAIR

*I*t is the traditional Japanese view that a serene mind, an active daily life, and an intelligent diet create the basics for skin beauty. The Japanese diet abounds in foods that are eaten for their medicinal, curative properties—foods that cleanse, balance, or strengthen the system.

The foods that are considered to be of particular benefit to the skin, either for their properties of purification or their strengthening, vitalizing actions, include sea plants, daikon radish, pearl barley, millet, Hokkaido pumpkin, wild Japanese parsley, black soybeans, azuki beans, buckwheat, perilla leaf, burdock root, miso, tofu, *natto,* cabbage, carrots, persimmons, celery, clams, oysters, sea urchins, cucumbers, spinach, tomatoes, green peppers, sesame seeds, and devil's tongue root. In the Japanese view, food is medicine—when a greasy, heavy, or spicy food is eaten, it is almost always accompanied by a food that will balance or neutralize the effects.

One of the simplest and most delightful ways to benefit from the traditional Japanese food-wisdom is to drink the easily prepared teas and broths which purify and vitalize the body, generating beauty from the inside. Many of the teas presented here may be taken as the internal counterpart to an external application of the same substance. This holistic approach to healthy beauty, the interconnected unity of inside and outside, is a basic premise of Asian herbal medicine. Because hair and skin benefit equally from many of the ingredients, teas used for both purposes are presented here.

Pearl Barley Tea

Actions:

Eliminates warts, freckles, and age spots
Lightens complexion
Eliminates toxins
Remedies pimples and rashes

Indications:

All skin types
Recommended for troubled skin
Take daily

Ingredients:

2 tablespoons (30 cc) pearl barley seeds
2 cups (480 ml) pure spring water

Preparation:

Roast the seeds by heating them in a heavy skillet over medium flame for 10 minutes, stirring constantly.

For the tea, add seeds to water in a nonmetal pan, bring to a boil, then lower the flame to simmer 10 minutes. Remove from the fire, steep 5 minutes, then strain to remove the seeds.

The tea may be stored in the refrigerator for 3 days.

Directions for Use:

Drink the tea hot or cold several times daily. The tea has diuretic properties, so it is important to consume adequate quantities of liquids, avoid overuse, and avoid giving it to children.

Pearl barley tea is Japan's most well-known and commonly prescribed internal complexion cure. A person who is serious about eliminating spots, freckles, warts, rashes—any type of imperfection or blemish—or lightening the skin will drink this tea daily, eat pearl barley in cream or porridge form, and apply pearl barley externally. Such a cure is said to bring results within one to three months.

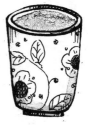

Tea Ceremony

Prepare tea with the deepest and fullest attention. Choose utensils, teapot, cup, and tea leaves for their beauty. Clean the utensils, the area for preparation, and the area for drinking with total attention to detail. Prepare a simple flower arrangement in a special vase, and place it where you will drink the tea. Slowly and softly and with grace of movement, boil the water. Place the tea leaves in the warmed teapot with reverence. Pour the water with consciousness into the pot. Sit quietly while the tea steeps. Pour it evenly and carefully into the cup. Hold the cup in your hands, feeling its warmth, noticing the beauty of the container. Respect the ancient tea leaf and appreciate its fragrance. Sip, taking in its warmth and delicate flavor. After drinking the tea, carefully clean the teapot, teacup, and utensils, and place them where they belong.

Pearl Barley Rice Cream

Actions:

As for pearl barley tea

Indications:

As for pearl barley tea

Ingredients:

1 tablespoon (15 cc) pearl barley seeds
1 tablespoon (15 cc) *mochiko* (flour made
   from *mochigome*—cooked glutinous rice)
Enough warm spring water to form a creamy
   mixture.

Preparation:

Grind the seeds to powder using a grain mill or
coffee-bean grinder, then mix the ingredients
together well, forming a cream.

Directions for Use:

Eat once daily over a prolonged period to
improve health and appearance of the skin.

*This very simple grain-and-seed
cream is eaten for only one
reason: to become more
beautiful.*

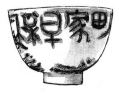

69

Black Bean Tea

Eaten as part of the first meal of the New Year, black beans are the symbolic representation of health. By stimulating the elimination of toxins, and thus purifying the blood, black bean tea is said to beautify the skin, giving it a rich luster and a translucent glow. Furthermore, black bean tea renders the drinker serene, a requirement of true beauty.

Actions:

Beautifies skin
Purifies blood
Stimulates circulation and metabolism
Warms
Calms

Indications:

Recommended for stressed or sluggish skin
Take once daily

Ingredients:

8 dried black soybeans
4¼ cups (1 liter) pure spring water
Sea salt

Preparation:

Boil the beans and water in a nonmetal pan until the volume of liquid is reduced by half. Add a pinch of sea salt and simmer for 1 to 2 minutes, then strain.

Directions for Use:

Drink a cup of black bean tea once daily.

Buckwheat Tea

Actions:

Beautifies skin
Strengthens system

Indications:

Recommended for lassitude
Take as desired

Ingredients:

2 teaspoons (10 cc) roasted, coarsely ground
  buckwheat kernels
1 cup (240 ml) pure spring water

Preparation:

(Roast buckwheat beforehand by heating in a
heavy skillet over medium high heat for 5
minutes, stirring. Grind very briefly so that the
kernels are in coarse chunks.)

Pour boiling water over the buckwheat to steep
in a teapot for 1 to 2 minutes.

Directions for Use:

Drink warm or cold.

Buckwheat tea has a nice smoky flavor; the fact that it is also a strengthener to the system and will make the skin glossy and supple makes this an altogether enchanting drink.

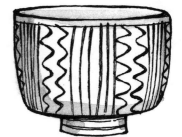

71

Pink Bean Tea

The shiny red azuki bean appears once again, this time incarnated as a beauty drink.

Actions:

Beautifies skin
Stimulates diuresis
Eliminates toxins
Combats stress
Helps prevent age spots

Indications:

Recommended for clearing the skin
Take once daily

Ingredients:

2 tablespoons (30 cc) pink bean powder
  of roasted azuki beans
1 cup (240 ml) pure spring water

(optional: 1 *umeboshi*—pickled plum)

Preparation:

Prepare azuki beans as for face-washing powder, by first roasting in a skillet, then grinding to a powder.

Stir the bean powder into just-boiled water and steep 5 minutes before drinking.

Another method is to boil the bean-water mixture for 5 minutes.

Directions for Use:

Drink warm. If accompanied by an *umeboshi*, the effect is particularly tonic and invigorating.

Simple Daikon Root Tea

Actions:

Stimulates diuresis
Eliminates toxins
Beautifies skin
Improves digestion

Indications:

Recommended for troubled skin (especially when
caused by eating the wrong foods)
Take once daily

Ingredients:

A slice of daikon (radish)
1 cup (240 ml) pure spring water
Sea salt

Preparation:

Grate the raw daikon with a daikon grater. Add
about 2 tablespoons (30 cc) of this to the water
with a pinch of salt, then bring to a boil for 1
to 2 minutes.

Directions for Use:

Allow the tea to cool slightly, then drink it.
Taken before a hot bath, this will encourage an
even more efficient elimination of toxins.

*It's common knowledge in Japan
that daikon is a purifier, and
it's used often for precisely this
reason. Raw and grated, it is
eaten with tempura to help the
body eliminate the extra oil.
Anyone who's feeling somewhat
poisoned by toxins or heavy rich
foods is likely to seek out the
refreshing, astringent, purifying
daikon. Girls are taught by their
mothers that raw daikon will
give them beautiful clear skin,
as white and translucent as the
daikon itself.*

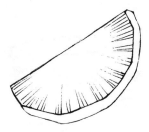

Burdock Root Tea

A very useful tea for women due to the high iron content, this is a beverage that will put color in your cheeks. I first learned about burdock root tea from my Yamagata midwife, who recommended it as a strengthening tea to be taken in late pregnancy, during labor, and also postpartum, to aid in healing and to tone the body. Burdock is also known for its beneficial effect on the reproductive systems of both men and women. It's said to improve men's sexual stamina.

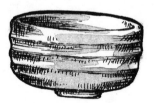

Actions:

Beautifies skin
Increases vitality
Eliminates wastes and toxins
Tones the system
Normalizes physiological functions

Indications:

Recommended for lack of color and tone
   in the skin
Take as often as desired

Ingredients:

4 ounces (120 cc) fresh burdock root, or
   2 ounces (60 cc) dried burdock root
2 cups (480 ml) pure spring water

Preparation:

Wash dirt from burdock root, but don't peel. Chop or julienne the root, then soak in cold water for 5 minutes. Bring burdock and water to a boil in a nonmetal pan, then simmer, covered, for 10 minutes. Strain to obtain liquid.

Directions for Use:

Drink in small amounts throughout the day. In one day, the total amount should not exceed 2 cups, as this tea is diuretic.

Saffron Tea

Actions:

Improves circulation
Prevents age spots and wrinkles
Beautifies hair

Indications:

Recommended for aging skin or poor circulation
Take occasionally

Ingredients:

3 pieces of saffron
1 cup (240 ml) pure spring water

Preparation:

Add the saffron to just-boiled hot water in a cup. Allow to sit for several minutes before drinking.

Directions for Use:

Sip the tea slowly.

Known as a woman's tea, helpful in improving the circulation and toning the female system, saffron tea is advised as a preventive tea against age spots. This is also a tea for the wealthy woman, as it is prohibitively expensive.

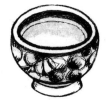

Seaweed Tea

This is a strangely delicate tea with a distinctive oceanic fragrance, something a sea goddess might sip.

Actions:

Eliminates toxins and fats
Beautifies hair and nails
Strengthens hair and revives color and shine

Indications:

Recommended for lifeless, dull, thin, falling, or graying hair
Take daily for 3 months or longer

Ingredients:

One strip of dried *kombu* seaweed, or 2 teaspoons (10 g) powdered *kombu*
2 cups (480 ml) pure spring water

Preparation:

If using dried *kombu*, boil in water for about 10 minutes.

Powdered *kombu* may simply be stirred into a cup of just-boiled water; use 1 teaspoon (5 g) per cup (240 ml). If desired, add a tiny strip of soft-boiled *kombu* to each cup before serving.

Directions for Use:

Drink as often as desired over a prolonged period.

Black Bean Tangerine Tea

Actions:

Beautifies hair and skin
Strengthens and tones

Indications:

Recommended for devitalized hair and skin
Take daily

Ingredients:

2 teaspoons (10 cc) black soybeans
1 teaspoon (5 cc) dried tangerine peel
2 cups (480 ml) pure spring water
Honey may be used for sweetening

Preparation:

Soak beans in water overnight. Bring beans, water, and tangerine peel to a boil in a nonmetal pan, then simmer for 5 minutes. Strain through cloth and add honey if desired for sweetening.

Directions for Use:

Drink warm.

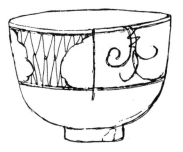

This drink is said to restore the natural color of hair going white, prevent hair loss, smooth and prevent wrinkles, lighten age spots, relieve stress, strengthen the kidneys and liver, improve digestion, invigorate the system, and make the body, skin, and hair more beautiful.

77

Miso Broth

One often hears, in regard to an elderly woman possessed of particularly fine white skin, "She must have eaten good miso every day of her life." Miso is good for skin, hair, and general health. While an instant miso broth may be made by stirring a tablespoon of miso paste into a cup of just-boiled water, the recipe given here offers the richer flavor and nourishment provided by a seaweed-fish stock.

Actions:

Nourishes
Beautifies skin and hair
Eliminates toxins
Aids digestion
Strengthens

Indications:

Recommended for devitalized hair and skin
Take daily

Ingredients:

1 small piece of *kombu* seaweed
1 cup (240 ml) pure water
1 tablespoon (15 cc) dried bonito flakes
1 tablespoon (15 cc) miso paste

Preparation:

Place *kombu* and water in a nonmetal pan and bring to a simmer. Remove *kombu* when boiling begins. Add bonito flakes while simmering, then remove from heat and steep 2 to 3 minutes. Filter to remove fish flakes, then add miso without cooking further.

Directions for Use:

Drink warm. May be reheated but not simmered again.

Black Sesame Kuzu Tea

Actions:

Prevents graying of hair
Nourishes hair
Darkens hair
Restores natural color
Gives luster and shine
Eliminates wrinkles and spots on the skin

Indications:

Recommended for lifeless, dull, thin, falling,
  graying hair
Take daily for 3 months or longer

Ingredients:

1 tablespoon (15 cc) black sesame seeds
2 tablespoons (30 cc) *kuzu* powder
1¼ cup (300 ml) pure spring water

Preparation:

Roast sesame seeds by heating over medium
flame for 1 to 2 minutes in a heavy skillet,
stirring constantly. They are ready when they
become aromatic.

Grind seeds using a mortar and pestle.

Mix *kuzu* and cold water in a nonmetal pan,
then cook over low flame until the mixture looks
thick and translucent. Add sesame and simmer
briefly while stirring.

The tea should be thick but easily poured. To
thin, add a little boiling water, stirring it in well.

Directions for Use:

Drink as is or with a little black sugar or honey.
This tea may be taken daily.

*The black-roasted sesame is
taken in Japan to darken the
hair, to prevent graying, and
even to bring back black hair
when the tresses turn white.
This sounds like magic, and
I don't know if it works,
but certain black-haired
Japanese grandmothers of my
acquaintance claim great
success with this method.*

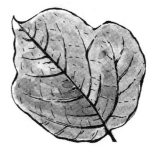

79

Sweet Ginger Kuzu Tea

The venerable root of kuzu is highly nourishing, easily digested, and medicinal. This kuzu drink acts as a nourishing, strengthening, stimulating tonic to the body. It will improve the circulation and generally set things right. This warming tea will also help prevent a cold from developing.

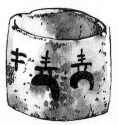

Actions:

Nourishes
Warms
Stimulates circulation
Strengthens
Combats illness

Indications:

Recommended for symptoms of fatigue, lifeless skin and hair
Take daily

Ingredients:

1 piece of ginger root
1 tablespoon (15 cc) black sugar or honey
1 teaspoon (5 cc) *kuzu* powder
1 cup (240 ml) pure spring water

Preparation:

Grate ginger and squeeze through cloth to obtain juice equivalent to 1 tablespoon. Dissolve *kuzu* in a little cold water, then add ginger juice and sweetener. Stir the rest of the water in, then simmer for a few minutes in a nonmetal pan, stirring constantly.

When the liquid thickens, it is ready.

Directions for Use:

Drink warm.

Cherry Bark Tea

Actions:

Beautifies hair
Encourages hair growth

Indications:

Recommended for thin hair
Take once daily

Ingredients:

1 teaspoon (5 cc) cherry bark
1 cup (240 ml) pure spring water

Preparation:

Place bark and water in a covered nonmetal pan and bring to a boil. Reduce heat to simmer until liquid is half the original volume. Steep covered for 5 minutes, then strain through cloth.

Directions for Use:

Drink hot.

Sit beneath a pink-blossoming cherry tree, watching the petals drift and float; drink tea made from the tree's bark; wait for your hair to grow long, long and longer. . . .

THE FACE-CARE RITUAL

Daily

Morning: Cleanse, first with oil, then with water-soluble cleansing substance.
Rinse, followed by a cold-water splash.
Apply water, rinse, or a tonic.
Apply an oil or emollient if desired.

Evening: Cleanse, first with oil, then with a water-soluble cleansing substance.
Use a warm-water rinse.
Massage with an oil or emollient.
Apply a water, rinse, or tonic if desired; an oil or emollient may be used as a nighttime treatment.

Weekly or as Needed

Morning or Evening: After cleansing and rinsing the face, apply a treatment, pack, or rub. Massage may precede such treatments, or in some cases the massage may be carried out using the same substance that will be used as a treatment pack. A rub can replace the usual facial massage. All treatments, packs, and rubs are designed to be followed by a warm-water rinse and then water, rinse, or a tonic. Only spot treatments like those applied to blemishes are not rinsed; these may be reapplied repeatedly throughout the day, as needed.

The teas may be incorporated into the daily regimen according to personal preference.

FACIAL REGIMENS

A personal facial regimen may be designed by choosing a la carte from among the recipes in each section. Select a cleansing oil, a wash, an oil for use in massage, a facial water or tonic, an oil for day or night use, a special treatment or pack, and a beauty tea, paying careful attention to your particular complexion needs and the indications given for each recipe. While most washes, waters, and oils may be used daily, the treatments and packs are designed for less frequent use. As many of the teas are medicinal, it is wise to take them no more frequently than directed. The following regimens suggest possible programs for some common complexion types and special needs.

Normal Skin
Camellia Cleansing Oil
Rice Bran Wash
Camellia Massage Oil
Loofah Vine Water
Camellia Day/Night Oil
Sea-Green Seaweed Pack
Buckwheat Tea

Sensitive Skin
Camellia Cleansing Oil
Pearl Barley and Pink Bean Powder Wash
Camellia Massage Oil
Ceremonial Green Tea Tonic
Camellia Day/Night Oil
Simple Tofu Pack
Pearl Barley Tea

Oily Skin
Sesame Cleansing Oil
Pink Bean Powder Wash
Aloe Massage Emollient
Ceremonial Green Tea Tonic
Aloe Day/Night Emollient
Whipped Egg-White Pack
Simple Daikon Root Tea

Young Skin
Honey and Walnut Cleansing Oil
Golden Honey Wash
Aloe Massage Emollient
First Water of Rice
Camellia Day/Night Oil
Japanese Honeysuckle Pack
Pearl Barley Tea

Dry Skin
Camellia Cleansing Oil
Rice Bran Wash
Shark's Liver Massage Oil
Black Sugar Rinse
Camellia Day Oil
Sesame Pack
Black Bean Tea

Aging Skin
Shark's Liver Cleansing Oil
Seaweed Scrub
Shark's Liver Massage Oil
Water of Pine
Camellia Day/Night Oil
Sea-Green Seaweed Pack
Buckwheat Tea

Blemished Skin
Black Sugar and Sesame Cleansing Oil
Pearl Barley and Pink Bean Powder Wash
(no massage)
Water of Lotus Root
Aloe Day/Night Emollient
Pearl Barley Tea
Pearl Barley Porridge Pack

Sunburned Skin
Sesame Cleansing Oil
Black Sugar Wash
(no massage)
Cucumber Juice Tonic
Aloe Day/Night Emollient
Summer Melon Pack
"Miso" Broth

To Lighten Skin
Black Sugar and Camellia Cleansing Oil
Pink Bean Powder Wash
Black Sugar and Camellia Massage Oil
Cucumber Juice Tonic
Camellia Day/Night Oil
Summer Melon Pack
Pearl Barley Tea

To Purify and Calm Stressed Skin
Camellia Cleansing Oil
Rice Bran Wash
Camellia Massage Oil
Water of Pine
Camellia Day/Night Oil
Three-Powder Pack
Pearl Barley Tea

To Revitalize Tired Skin
Black Sugar and Camellia Cleansing Oil
Black Sugar Wash
Black Sugar and Sesame Massage Oil
Pink Plum Sake
Camellia Day/Night Oil
Sea-Green Seaweed Pack
Burdock Root Tea

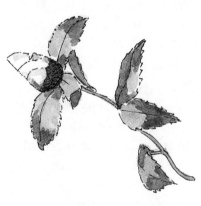

To live in poetic harmony with the seasons of nature, use the following regimens:

Autumn
Walnut Cleansing Oil
Rice Bran Wash
Walnut Massage Oil
Water of Lotus Root
Walnut Day/Night Oil
October Persimmon Pack
Burdock Root Tea

Spring
Camellia Cleansing Oil
Pink Bean Powder Wash
Honey and Camellia Massage Oil
Ceremonial Green Tea Tonic
Camellia Day/Night Oil
Pink Bean Powder Pack
Pink Bean Tea

Winter
Sesame Cleansing Oil
Black Sugar Wash
Sesame Massage Oil
Water of Pine
Sesame Day/Night Oil
Winter Salad Face Pack
Black Bean Tea

Summer
Safflower Cleansing Oil
Pink Bean Powder Wash
Safflower Massage Oil
Pink Plum Sake
Safflower Day/Night Oil
Summer Melon Pack
Iced Pearl Barley Tea

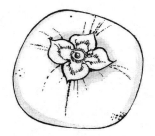

PART TWO
THE BEAUTY OF THE HAIR

THE BEAUTY OF THE HAIR

Hair is a great natural resource of Japan—it grows strong, thick, straight as a waterfall, blue-black and shiny. This natural wealth is maintained by: a strengthening diet, full of foods eaten specifically to nourish, protect, and enrich the hair's beauty and health; the scalp massage, including pressure-point stimulation to benefit circulation and metabolism; the scrupulous protection of the hair and head from sun damage; the careful, gentle grooming and handling of the hair in styling; the application of gentle shampoos; and nourishing, protective rinses and treatments to strengthen hair externally.

In Japan, where the refined response to beauty has been developed to a kind of apogee, beautiful hair on a woman is understood as something provocative, evoking an immediate visceral response in the masculine viewer. By the beauty of her hair alone, goes the saying, a woman can captivate a man.

The realm of women's hair is one of the few where the Japanese depart from the minimal "small is beautiful," "less is more" approach. For centuries, Japanese women wore their hair as long as possible; to cut the hair was considered an act of extreme sacrifice, practiced by those entering into Buddhist nunhood or those mourning a departed husband. The longer the hair, the more evocative its suggestion of nature and sensuality. Though long, feminine hair gave way to modern, practical, shorter haircuts after the turn of the century, the ideal Japanese beauty is always a woman with long, black, straight hair.

Perfectly groomed hair was and remains the Japanese standard. To have just one wisp of hair out of place—like the accidentally revealed flash of white leg seen under the all-enveloping kimono—supplies the subtlest, therefore most intense, of erotic hints. That such stray wisps and accidental glimpses may be artfully contrived is of no importance—what matters is that they suggest accident. To be effective, such details must be small, on the verge of nonexistent.

Healthy hair is hair that is naturally beautiful, rich in color, smooth and shiny. With such hair as a starting point, one may then proceed to dress it with fragrant oils and ornament and arrange it with elegance, remembering to permit the straying of the tiniest, faintest, accidental wisp.

THE JAPANESE SHAMPOO

Ten centuries ago, during the Heian era, when beautiful women wore their black hair draped long to the floor, when their hair fell thick, straight, and heavy from a middle part like a mysterious silken curtain, washing the hair was hard work. Special days were set aside for the task: at Kyoto's Kamo River, for example, the seventh of July was the day for that month's shampoo. During the Heian era, there were entire periods when washing one's hair was forbidden—the taboo months were April, May, September, and October.

In Japan as in other parts of the world, the shampoo has been historically an infrequent ritual until relatively recent times. In the Meiji era, it was the custom to shampoo one's hair approximately once monthly, with a gradual increase in frequency as hairstyles and aesthetic standards changed; the modern Japanese woman shares the same zeal for the almost-daily shampoo that is seen worldwide these days.

Until this century, the substances used for washing the hair in Japan were those that had been favored for centuries: camellia oil, seaweed, eggs, rice bran,

---

Steps in the Japanese shampoo

- Carried out as part of the prebath washing ritual, the bather sits on the bathstool or kneels, inclining the head so that the hair falls forward. The hair is moistened with warm water.
- Follow specific instructions given for each shampoo. In general, shampoo is applied to the scalp and not to the hair ends directly.
- Thoroughly massage the scalp for 5 minutes or so, pressing firmly with the fingertips of both hands and performing very small rotations or side-to-side movements—moving the scalp and not displacing the fingertips—over the entire scalp. Avoid pulling, scratching, tugging, or any rough handling of the hair.
- To cleanse the hair, gently smooth and pat the hair ends, allowing the shampoo liquid to disperse throughout the hair. The hair is never scrubbed or pulled, but handled with as much delicacy as if it were a length of fine silk.
- To rinse, shower the head with tepid water, with the hair still held in the forward-falling position, rinsing for as long as possible to remove all traces of shampoo.

---

and bean powder. These natural washes were followed by botanical rinses to purify and tone, with oils, pomades, or plant juices applied for styling the hair, and an occasional incense-smoking treatment for hair fragrance.

The Japanese shampoo is perhaps best thought of as a cleansing massage. Traditional wisdom puts the emphasis on the scalp massage and gives cleansing a place of lesser importance. To remove all oil from the hair is thought to leave it defenseless, dry, and vulnerable to breakage.

In earlier times, the poorest farmers and villagers used natural clay as a shampoo, which was a very efficient cleanser, but stripped the hair so completely that it became dry, lost its deep black color to become reddish or brownish, and even grew frizzy or wavy. Those who used the bran-rich water from rice-washing fared better, due to rice bran's generous moisturizing and nourishing properties, while the upper-class wives of samurai and aristocrats used mineral-laden sea plants, and gloried in hair that was glossy, black, and thick.

None of the natural Japanese shampoos described here strip the hair of its oils. These hair washes do cleanse the hair of dirt, nourish and stimulate the hair and scalp, and leave the hair gently moisturized. The traditional Japanese shampoo strikes a fine balance between purification and protection, with the thorough scalp massage providing stimulation of the circulation and relaxation of tension. (A head massage properly executed will stimulate the pressure points as well, bringing toning, regenerating benefits to one's total being.)

Crushed Camellia Nut Shampoo

Actions:

Cleanses slightly
Protects
Moisturizes
Nourishes scalp and hair
Improves texture and condition

Indications:

Recommended for dry or damaged hair
Weekly use

Ingredients:

Nuts from the camellia tree

Preparation:

Place 30 nuts in a large scrubbing bag, tied tightly with a cord. Strike the bag repeatedly against a hard surface to shatter the nuts and cause the emergence of camellia oil.

Directions for Use:

Rub the bag thoroughly and gently over the scalp and unmoistened hair. The movement of the strokes must be as for brushing—from the roots of the hair to the ends. This is a "dry" shampoo, so no use of water is required.

Because this technique leaves hair oiled, it may be most appreciated by those with very thick or very curly hair—hair that is fine or thin will seem lank.

Modern women of many cultures are in the habit of shampooing daily, then inundating their heads with conditioners, treatment creams, rinses, serums, and balms to give hair body, texture, and shine. A simpler method was followed in earlier times: women not only washed their hair much less frequently, but often nourished and styled it with the use of oil. Their hair was undoubtedly very healthy, if aesthetically unappealing by present standards.

The Japanese Crushed Camellia Nut Shampoo is an ancient ancestor of the many camellia shampoos now produced in Japan. The friend who described the shampoo method to me said, "First you crash the bag to crush the nuts."

Rice Bran Shampoo

The honorable grain of rice! It beautifies not only the landscape, with glistening gold-green vistas of late-summer rice fields, but also the meal-table, with steaming bowls of fragrant white, and with the nourishing, polishing bran, bringing a soft gleam to the wooden floors of houses, women's skin, and women's long, long hair. This shampoo is cleanser and conditioner in one, used on beautiful Japanese hair for centuries.

92

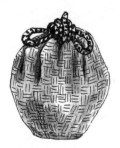

Actions:

Cleanses
Moisturizes

Indications:

All hair types
Use as needed

Ingredients:

Fresh pure rice bran
or
Water used for washing rice

Directions for Use:

If using rice bran, fill a cotton or silk bag, soak in warm water, then massage scalp and hair gently with the bag, remoistening it as necessary. Rinse.

If using the water from rice-washing, place the milky liquid in a basin, then pour repeatedly over the head, catching the runoff in the basin. Massage the scalp and rub the liquid through the hair thoroughly. Rinse.

Pink Bean Powder and Olive Oil Shampoo

Actions:

Cleanses
Moisturizes

Indications:

All hair types
Use as needed

Ingredients:

Pure virgin olive oil
Pink powder of azuki

Directions for Use:

Apply a small amount of olive oil to the hair and scalp, massaging well and making sure some oil reaches the ends of the hair.

Azuki bean powder is then applied dry to the hair, rubbed in gently and completely, and rinsed.

This is followed by applying azuki powder that has been mixed with warm water, massaging well once again, then a final thorough rinsing.

NOTE: For those who do not care for the softly oiled texture of hair after this shampoo (which is very good for the hair!) a small amount of commercial shampoo may be used with the azuki powder.

When, in the course of my research into the ancient beauty traditions of Japan, I kept encountering olive oil, I was puzzled. Though one now and then notices a minuscule curve of olive on a contemporary Japanese pizza, it would certainly be a rare and momentous occasion if an olive were to make an appearance at an average Japanese meal. The olive is exotic in Japan, so how on earth did the old-fashioned beauties discover its benefits to hair and skin? Then, looking at a time line of Japanese history one day, I remembered the Portuguese. They came to Japan in 1542, bringing Christianity, guns, a cake called kasutera, and quite possibly, I conjectured, olive oil. At any rate, whatever its origin, virgin olive oil is highly regarded as a beauty treatment for skin and hair. Like camellia oil, it's a trusted Japanese classic.

Sea Tangle Shampoo

The upper-class wives of samurai used seaweed shampoo, and it was said that this was the source of their strong, shining, beautiful black hair. Like all the Japanese cleansing methods, seaweed not only removes dirt and excess oil, but imparts a rich supply of nutrients, leaving hair lustrous, thick, and easy to arrange. The deep-sea aroma can be heady; women of old Japan used so much water to rinse their seaweed-washed heads that public baths charged higher rates for women bathers.

Actions:

Cleanses
Nourishes
Gives volume and luster

Indications:

All hair types
Use as needed

Ingredients:

1 teaspoon (5 cc) powdered dried sea plants (*kombu, funori,* and *hijiki* is a good combination)
¾ cup (180 ml) pure spring water

Preparation:

Dried seaweed may be powdered in a blender or food processor. The powder can be stored in a jar in a dry location.

Fresh seaweed must be washed and soaked for 10 to 20 minutes to eliminate salt. The seaweed can then be pureed in a blender or with a mortar and pestle for immediate use. Fresh seaweed puree cannot be stored, though it may be refrigerated for a day or two. It is preferable to make a fresh batch for each shampoo.

Directions for Use:

Mix the seaweed powder or puree with warm water in a teacup, stirring until the mixture is creamy. This can be done several hours prior to shampooing, but no later than 30 minutes beforehand.

When the mixture is ready, wet the hair and apply to scalp and hair. Massage gently and thoroughly before rinsing. (This shampoo may be left on the head for 20 minutes or so as a pack if desired.)

An alternative method, for those who prefer the squeaky-clean shampoo feeling, is to precede the seaweed shampoo with a wash using one's usual shampoo, or to mix a little commercial shampoo with the seaweed—in which case the mixture should not be left on as a pack.

Rinse extremely well, and if desired, add a teaspoon of rice vinegar to the final rinse, to eliminate oceanic aromas.

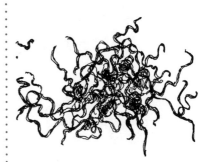

Violet Seaweed Shampoo

My daughter loves this shampoo because it's plum-pink and comes from the beach— something baby mermaids would use. Funori is a curly red-violet seaweed with little pods that pop delightfully when pinched. Sold in Japan for use in cooking and as a laundry starch, funori makes a gluey mucilage that some people use in small amounts as a setting gel. As a shampoo, funori is extraordinary—hair feels silky, luxuriant, thick and nourished, with a lovely obedience to styling.

Actions:

Cleanses
Nourishes
Gives volume and shine

Indications:

All hair types
Use as needed

Ingredients:

Handful of dried *funori*
3 cups (710 ml) pure spring water

Preparation:

Place *funori* in a nonmetal pan with water, bring to a boil, then remove from heat and allow to cool. Filter the liquid through a cloth or sieve, discarding the seaweed solids.

Directions for Use:

Apply the pink gel to wet hair and massage into the scalp and hair. The substance may be left on the hair for 20 minutes or so as a pack if desired.

Rinse thoroughly. Add a tablespoon of rice vinegar to the last rinse to eliminate the sea fragrance.

Whipped Egg-White "Dry" Shampoo

Actions:

Cleanses
Softens

Indications:

All hair types
Use as needed

Ingredients:

Whipped egg white

Preparation:

Whip the white of an egg (two, if your hair is long) until stiff, as for meringue.

Directions for Use:

Used as a "dry" shampoo, the whipped egg white is applied to dry hair and massaged into the scalp, then removed by wiping repeatedly with a towel that has been dipped in hot water and wrung out.

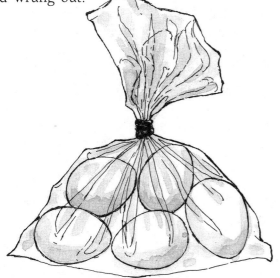

This is one of the very old-time hair cleansers. It must have come in handy during all those months of tabooed shampoos. But how many egg whites might be required by a floor-length head of hair?

THE SCALP MASSAGE FOR HAIR BEAUTY

The basic head massage, carried out attentively and applied to every part of the scalp, will stimulate both pressure points and the circulation of the scalp, with the reward of a beautiful, healthy head of hair. The massage should be practiced daily, in conjunction with shampoo or treatment application, or at any time that is convenient. The following points should be observed: The scalp should be warm—during a shampoo or after a hot bath are good times. After moistening the hair with very warm water and applying shampoo or a treatment substance, the scalp should be massaged by first placing all ten fingers so that the two hands meet finger to finger along the center-part line.

From that starting point, begin by pressing and making very small rotations with all the fingertips (not the nails), gradually moving downward, moving the scalp and not the fingers over the scalp. The same vigorous technique is applied to every part of the scalp. Points which feel particularly loose, tender, or tight are said to be an indication of an energy blockage or imbalance somewhere in the body—if not in the head itself—and should receive extra attention.

Another technique for scalp massage involves the use of a comb or brush. While for grooming the hair a comb is the utensil of choice, for stimulating the scalp a natural-bristle brush is a useful tool. The important thing to remember is that it is the *scalp* and not the hair which is being brushed, and when moving the brush through the hair great care must be taken to proceed with delicacy. If a comb is used, it should be a Japanese boxwood comb or a very good blunt-toothed rubber one. A brush should have rounded bristles.

The brushing-massage technique is as follows: Place the brush at the very top of the head, directly up from the ears at the very center of the head. This is the starting point for each stroke. From this point, first stroke down toward the forehead, next to the temples, then to the ears, then toward the edges of the hairline at the neck. The brush or comb is moved very slowly and carefully, applied directly and firmly to the scalp.

In this brush-massage, hair is brushed away from that one central point in a radial manner, never all forward or all back, as one might usually do when brushing the hair.

For the following technique, the same brush or a smaller one may be used, preferably one with rounded natural bristles which have some stiffness: The brush is to be applied firmly to each part of the head, pressed for three- to five-second periods, repeating the pressure at each spot five times. A final specialized technique consists of applying the brush to an area where hair is graying: while applying firm pressure, move the brush ever so slightly back and forth against the spot without pulling at the hair or causing it stress of any kind. This technique, like the others, moves the scalp and not the brush upon the scalp. This treatment is not advisable for areas of thinning hair.

Other treatments which will benefit the look and health of the hair take place at the other end of the body: the feet. The split-bamboo foot-treader, a foot massage, or even a very hot footbath are all advised as remedies for poor circulation in the head area.

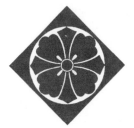

HAIR RINSES AND TREATMENTS

*B*ecause Japanese women traditionally washed their hair infrequently, and then only with gentle, nourishing, natural substances, followed by the application of oils or plant juices for dressing the hair, a postshampoo conditioning rinse was not necessary. At no point was the hair stripped of natural oils, as it is with today's efficient chemical shampoos that render it vulnerable to dehydration, sun damage, and tangling.

Oil and plant extracts combed through the hair during the styling process served to control the hair and also to supply protection; most hairdressing oils contained essential oils, offering not only a variety of healing, nourishing, or stimulating properties, but acting as natural antiseptics that purify the hair and scalp as well.

Special treatments and rinses were applied to remedy specific conditions: falling hair, dandruff, scalp irritations, or loss of color or shine. Many of the botanical substances used for bathing or for treating the skin also benefit the hair; when a curative beauty regimen is undertaken, many of the substances may be used both externally and internally for best results. Seaweed, camellia nut oil, eggs, ginger root, garlic, *sake,* black sugar, and a variety of fruits, leaves, grains, and seeds all offer beauty and health to the hair, whether used for curative or merely protective purposes.

While rinses, treatments, and oils can be of enormous benefit to the hair, offering stimulation, toning, nourishment, shine, purification, and protection against moisture loss and damage, the hair must be guarded from the elements to maintain its beauty. Sunlight can be as damaging to the hair as it is to the skin, and the head should be shielded from overexposure whenever possible. Every visitor to Japan immediately notices the plethora of hats—hats worn by women, babies, and young children in the outdoor sunshine to protect both skin and hair from damage. Farm women wrap *tenugui* cloths around their heads for the same reason, or even more commonly, wear broad-brimmed straw hats with attached scarves that cover the delicate skin of the neck and face as completely as possible. In the summertime in towns and cities, women protected under white parasols can be seen everywhere.

Another important element in the protection of hair beauty is gentle handling. Many modern experts agree with the traditional Japanese wisdom: Hair should be combed with a good comb, but never brushed. The stimulation of the scalp and the distribution of hair oils through the tresses which many associate with brushing may be better achieved by gentle combing and scalp massage. Brushing the hair can have a harsh effect on the cuticle, causing breakage and splitting unless executed with infinite delicacy. The damage caused by the overuse or incorrect use of heated styling tools or blow dryers is well known, as is the drying effect caused by many styling mousses, sprays, and gels. To dispense with these things entirely is preferable.

The treatments and rinses described here fall into the following categories: the postshampoo conditioning rinse, the preshampoo treatment pack, the post-shampoo treatment pack, and special treatments, usually oils or plant juices which are meant to be applied to the scalp or hair and left there as an all-day or all-night treatment.

How to apply the Japanese hair rinses and treatments

- The Postshampoo Conditioning Rinse is applied to just-shampooed hair, after all shampoo has been rinsed from the hair. Some rinses are designed to be poured repeatedly over the head, while for others once is enough. Some rinses act as the final rinse, while others must be followed by a clear-water rinse.
- The Preshampoo Treatment Pack is applied to wet or dry hair prior to shampooing. Because the scalp is more responsive to treatment substances when pores are dilated and the skin is warm and relaxed, during a bath soak is a good time to apply such a pack. To remove the pack, first rinse with copious amounts of warm water, then apply shampoo and wash well, rinse, and follow up with a light conditioning rinse if desired.
- The Postshampoo Treatment Pack is applied after shampooing and rinsing the hair. The pack is applied to the scalp and hair for the specified length of time and then rinsed for at least five minutes with clear tepid water. No further shampooing or conditioning is needed.
- The Special Treatment is generally applied to dry hair, massaged into the scalp somewhat, and then left for a prolonged period, either around the clock or only at night, depending on the recipe and personal preference. The special treatments are usually designed as long-term regimens.
- Note that the scalp massage may be carried out at any point in the hair-care ritual: during the shampoo, while applying a treatment or a rinse to wet hair, or while applying a special treatment to dry hair.

SPECIAL TREATMENTS

While most of the shampoos, packs, and rinses are hair health and beauty treatments in themselves, there are a few special curative treatments that may be required when hair is severely damaged, breaking excessively, falling out, or otherwise behaving particularly badly.

Onion and **garlic** are both used in Japan to treat female hair loss. The raw juice of either is applied daily to the affected area; this regimen is followed for two or three months. Warming the spot with a steamed towel before applying juice is said to improve the scalp's responsiveness to the treatment. Because hair so readily takes on any kind of fragrance, it is hard to imagine anyone but a hermitess following this program. An alternative approach to consider: apply odorless garlic oil, available in gelatin capsules, instead.

Sesame oil and **camellia oil**, a few drops massaged daily into the scalp, are said to help prevent hair loss and improve the hair's general condition, including color. Before applying heat to the hair with a blow-dryer, or before using any chemical agent, a little oil may be massaged into damp hair for protection. Intense cold and wind, extreme heat, or bright sunshine will be less likely to damage the hair if these oils are applied before exposure. The best time to apply the oil is after a shampoo or a bath-soak, when the hair is damp and the scalp is warm. A gentle combing after the hair is dry will help the oil to reach all areas.

Another way to use camellia oil is to apply a scant drop or two to dry hair, followed by a drop or two of **lemon** juice, both of which are said to be healing and restorative substances for the hair, particularly when used together.

Traditional hair treatments for protection from damage by sun or cold were, along with those already mentioned, a mixture of either **castor oil** and camellia oil or castor oil and *shochu*, the high-proof Japanese distilled spirits for which vodka may be substituted. Castor oil is a healing oil that is said to stimulate hair growth as well as protect the hair and give it gloss, but it is very heavy, an oily oil, so this treatment is difficult to adapt for modern use, unless one favors the greased wet look. As a nighttime treatment, castor oil may be massaged into the scalp and combed through the hair, concentrating on dry or damaged ends. Regarding the *shochu*-oil treatment, the mixture would seem useful as a purifying, antiseptic remedy, but it is likely that the alcohol would be drying if overused.

Soybean Tea

Actions:

Enriches
Nourishes

Indications:

All hair types
Recommended for scalp irritations, tired hair
Use daily or as desired

Ingredients:

1¾ ounces (50 cc) dried soybeans
2 cups (480 ml) pure spring water

Preparation:

Prepare a decoction by bringing the soybeans and water to a boil in a nonmetal pan, then reduce heat and simmer until the liquid is reduced by half.

Keeping the pan covered, steep the tea until it is cool. Filter through a cloth.

The soybean tea will last up to 3 days if refrigerated.

Directions for Use:

Apply liquid to hair after shampooing as a conditioning rinse. Subsequent clear-water rinsing is not necessary.

NOTE: This tea can be used for basic daily care.

The plebeian little soybean, so nourishing when eaten or used externally, offers the hair a rich cocktail of protein, B vitamins, and minerals. For dry hair, an occasional soybean oil massage will further increase the benefits of the bean-tea conditioner.

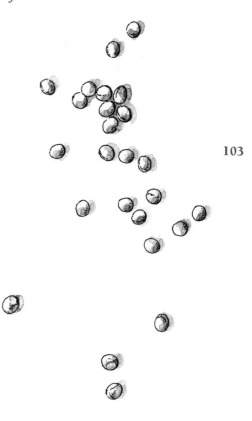

First Water of Rice Rinse

The glorious rice grain is at the spiritual center of Japanese culture; as befits such a beloved staple food, it may be found in every phase of the natural beauty ritual.

Actions:

Moisturizes
Nourishes
Gives shine

Indications:

All hair types
Recommended for dry or damaged hair
Use as often as desired

Ingredients:

One filled rice-bran bag
Pure spring water

Preparation:

Place the rice-bran bag in a nonmetal pan with twice the amount of water, then bring to a boil, lower heat, and simmer for 15 minutes. Allow to cool, then remove the rice-bran bag.

Prepare fresh for each use.

Directions for Use:

After shampooing, apply as a conditioning rinse, leaving on the hair for a few minutes, then rinsing with clear water.

NOTE: This rinse can be used for basic daily care.

Brown Rice Vinegar Rinse

Actions:

Purifies
Nourishes
Balances
Tones
Helps eliminate product buildup
Revives

Indications:

All hair types
Use as needed or after each shampoo

Ingredients:

1 tablespoon (15 ml) brown rice vinegar
1 cup (240 ml) warm water

Preparation:

Mix vinegar into the water.

Directions for Use:

After shampooing the hair and rinsing thoroughly, use the vinegar-water as the final rinse for the hair.

NOTE: This rinse can be used for basic daily care.

Rice appears again, this time in sweet-sour vinegar form—a light refreshment for the hair.

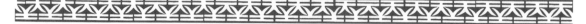

Camellia Water Rinse

Along with its atmosphere of strong-but-delicate feminine spirit, camellia oil has another more mysterious magic; it is said to bestow long life and youth to people—an ancient Chinese belief—and to restore freshness and flavor to old rice. The oil is protective, as are all oils, but it has a certain refreshing quality not usually associated with oil.

Actions:

Nourishes
Smooths
Softens
Moisturizes
Eliminates tangles

Indications:

All hair types
Use as needed

Ingredients:

2 to 3 drops of camellia nut oil
4¼ cups (1 liter) warm spring water

Preparation:

Mix the oil with the water well, making sure that the oil is dispersed in the water.

Directions for Use:

After shampooing and rinsing the hair, pour the camellia water rinse over the head.

NOTE: This rinse can be used for basic daily care.

106

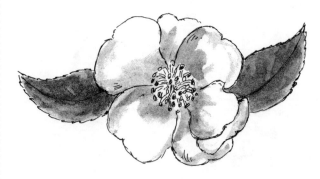

Licorice Root Tea Rinse

Actions:

Smooths
Softens
Revives

Indications:

All hair types
Recommended for unmanageable or frizzy hair
Use daily or as desired

Ingredients:

2 ounces (60 cc) powdered or chopped licorice
   root
2½ cups (600 ml) pure spring water

Preparation:

Bring ingredients to a boil in a nonmetal pan,
then lower heat and simmer for 30 minutes. Add
water to bring the final volume to 1¼ cups
(300 ml), then cool at room temperature and
filter through gauze.

The mixture will keep refrigerated for up to 3
days.

Directions for Use:

Use as a conditioning rinse after shampooing. A
clear-water rinse is not required.

NOTE: This rinse can be used for basic daily care.

*Licorice root, sweeter than sugar
and internally soothing as a
medicinal, tonic tea, is the sweet
remedy for frizzy, flyaway hair.
Known as kanzou in Japan, it
is Glycyrrhiza glabra in Latin.*

107

Camellia Oil Treatment

If one's toilette consisted only of rice bran and camellia oil, with perhaps a little sake as well, one could easily and elegantly accomplish all aspects of the beauty ritual.

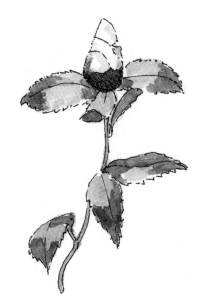

Actions:

Nourishes hair and scalp
Moisturizes
Alleviates dandruff
Prevents color fading
Prevents breakage and hair loss

Indications:

All hair types
Use weekly

Ingredients:

Camellia nut oil

Directions for Use:

Before shampooing the hair, brush the hair gently as described in the section on scalp massage. Apply camellia oil to scalp and hair, massaging the scalp well and spreading oil throughout the hair, concentrating on damaged ends.

Wrap head in a warm towel, then leave on for as long as possible (30 minutes to 3 hours).

Rinse hair with very warm water, then shampoo well and rinse.

NOTE: Use as an occasional treatment or for special conditions.

Sesame Oil Treatment

Actions:

Prevents hair loss
Nourishes hair and scalp
Heals
Moisturizes

Indications:

Recommended for dry, damaged, dull, or
thinning hair
Use weekly

Ingredients:

Sesame oil

Directions for Use:

Before shampooing the hair, apply sesame oil to
slightly moistened hair, massaging the scalp
thoroughly and oiling the hair itself all the way
to the ends. Wrap the head in a warm towel,
and leave the oil on the head for at least 30
minutes, or as long as 3 hours.

Rinse with very warm water, then shampoo the
hair well and rinse.

**NOTE: Use as an occasional treatment or for special
conditions.**

*Used as the carrier oil in
traditional scented hair oil and
as a fundamental ingredient in
Asian herbal medicine, sesame
oil is the one used most often
for healing purposes where hair
and scalp are concerned. A
sesame regimen for hair health
involves the external application
and massage with the oil,
combined with the daily
consumption of sesame seeds as
a condiment, in white or black,
raw or toasted form.*

109

Garlic Rice Wine

For luxuriant, glossy, well-nourished, soft and smooth, garlic-scented tresses.

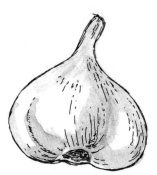

Actions:

Stimulates scalp circulation
Prevents hair loss
    and breakage
Alleviates dandruff
Protects

Indications:

Not recommended for sensitive scalps
Recommended for tired, damaged, dull, or
    breaking hair

Ingredients:

6 garlic cloves
2 cups (480 ml) *sake* (rice wine)
(Optional: camellia or sesame oil)

Preparation:

Heat *sake* until it is almost boiling, then remove from heat and add peeled, halved garlic cloves to the liquid. Cover and allow to steep for 30 minutes or longer. (Stored in the refrigerator, the liquid will keep for some time, but is best used within a week or so.)

Directions for Use:

Before shampooing, apply the liquid to hair and scalp, massaging thoroughly and spreading the liquid completely through the hair. Wrap head in warm towel and leave for 30 minutes, then rinse with warm water, shampoo, and rinse again.

NOTE: Use as an occasional treatment or for special conditions.

Sesame Oil With Ginger

Actions:

Stimulates hair growth
Remedies falling hair
Heals scalp irritations
Alleviates dandruff
Activates circulation

Indications:

Not recommended for sensitive scalps
Recommended for tired hair, falling hair
Use as desired, as a prolonged cure, three times weekly

Ingredients:

Fresh ginger root
Sesame oil

Preparation:

Grate a piece of ginger root with a ginger grater, then squeeze in a piece of gauze. Discard solids, and save ginger juice to mix in a 1:1 ratio with pure sesame oil, beating well with a whisk.

Prepare fresh for each use.

Directions for Use:

Use as a massage oil for the scalp, rubbing into the head and hair roots for 10 minutes prior to shampooing.

This oil may also be left on the head as a pack treatment, though some skins may be irritated by ginger. If there is any stinging sensation, wash the oil from the hair at once, and decrease the quantity of ginger in future mixtures.

NOTE: Use as an occasional treatment or for special conditions.

Though this treatment will leave you smelling faintly of an aromatic Chinese kitchen, it is used to stimulate hair growth and alleviate a hair loss problem, so perhaps this noble aim can justify the somewhat pungent fragrance.

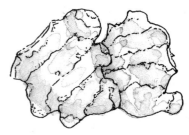

111

Honey Citron Rice Wine

A friend of mine tells me that she has become sake-crazed, applying sake to hair and skin, pouring it by the liter into her hot bath; it all started when her husband brought home a cheap jar of "cup" sake, the kind sold in vending machines all over Japan, and told her about his beautiful, fresh-faced grandmother and how all she used for beauty was rice wine. My friend does not do anything halfway, so she diligently sampled hundreds of grades and varieties of sake before coming to the conclusion that the cheapest sake is the best.

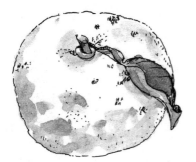

Actions:

Alleviates dandruff
Purifies
Invigorates

Indications:

Recommended for dandruff or tired hair
Use twice weekly

Ingredients:

Juice from 1 *yuzu* (citron) or lemon
1 tablespoon (15 ml) honey
2 tablespoons (30 ml) *sake* (rice wine)

Preparation:

Mix the ingredients together well.

Directions for Use:

Before shampooing the hair, apply the treatment pack to dry or slightly moistened hair. Allow to remain for 5 to 20 minutes before rinsing and washing the hair.

NOTE: This treatment can be used for basic daily care.

Seaweed Tea Rinse

Actions:

Nourishes
Tones
Stimulates
Softens

Indications:

All hair types
Use as needed

Ingredients:

2 strips dried *kombu* (kelp) seaweed
¾ cup (180 ml) pure spring water

Preparation:

Boil water and pour over the seaweed in a nonmetal container, then allow to sit for 30 minutes or until the seaweed is soft. Remove the seaweed before using.

Directions for Use:

After shampooing and rinsing the hair, pour seaweed tea over the hair and massage for several minutes before rinsing with tepid water.

NOTE: This rinse can be used for basic daily care.

Enrich hair with a light green broth of hot-steeped ocean kelp.

Black Sugar Syrup Treatment Pack

Just as enriching to the hair as it is to the skin, black sugar will nourish and strengthen the hair with a concentrated dose of minerals. Those with dry or dull hair may combine the syrup with sesame or camellia oil, in which case the shampoo afterward must be very thorough.

Actions:

Nourishes

Tones

Indications:

All hair types

Recommended for damaged hair

Use occasionally

Ingredients:

Black sugar syrup (see chapter on face washes)

Directions for Use:

Apply black sugar syrup or black sugar diluted in a small amount of hot water to the hair as a postshampoo pack. Wrap the head in a warm towel and allow to remain for 20 minutes. A soak in the bath at the same time will provide the proper warm and steamy atmosphere.

If oil is used, the pack must be applied before shampooing, and hair must be carefully washed to remove most oil.

NOTE: Use as an occasional treatment or for special conditions.

Egg-Yolk Treatment Pack

Actions:

Cleanses
Thickens
Nourishes
Moisturizes

Indications:

Recommended for dry or damaged hair
Use once or twice weekly

Ingredients:

One or two fresh egg yolks

Preparation:

Beat yolks slightly with a whisk.

For a more appealing fragrance my variation on the egg-yolk treatment is to add a drop or two of essential oil. The traditional Japanese scents are sandalwood, clove, and fennel, all of which lend a pleasant perfume to the hair.

Directions for Use:

This treatment is applied after shampooing the hair, as a pack to be left on for 10 to 20 minutes, then rinsed well for at least 5 minutes.

NOTE: Use as an occasional treatment or for special conditions.

The egg is an international thing, knowing no cultural boundaries. As one of the richest of hair nourishers, the egg belongs to the Japanese beauty tradition and undoubtedly all traditions everywhere. The egg gives to long hair a splendid undulation.

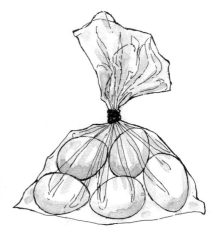

BEAUTY FOODS

If one wished to design a simple, nutritious, low-calorie meal that would ensure stunningly beautiful, luxuriant hair, one might end up with something like this:

A Whole Grain
A Small Portion of Grilled Fish
or
A Raw Egg
Sea Plants
A Soybean Product
Seeds or Nuts

This meal, abundant in all the B vitamins, high in low-fat protein, brimming with hair-beautifying minerals like sulphur, iron, and zinc, along with plenty of calcium and vegetable oils, is light, filling, and when eaten regularly over an extended period, is absolutely guaranteed to make beautiful, strong, shiny, thick hair. This meal is the basic everyday Japanese breakfast (with one important adjustment: while the Japanese customarily eat white rice or at best rice with the germ still intact, there is no doubt that whole rice is the superior food):

Brown Rice Sprinkled with Sesame Seeds
Grilled Fish
and/or
A Raw Egg
Miso Soup with *Wakame* Seaweed and Tofu
Toasted *Nori* Seaweed
Natto Fermented Soybeans

This simple meal—everything is eaten is small quantities—is beautifying and health-giving not only to the hair, but to the skin and one's entire physical being. Further, the *umeboshi* pickle which is almost always included serves to facilitate digestion and purify the body of toxins—a medicinal tonic that strengthens and vitalizes all body functions.

Truly beautiful hair requires not only cleansing, stimulation and massage of the scalp, the protection and nourishment offered by gentle, enriching washes, rinses, and treatments, gentleness in handling and protection from the elements—icy winds, dry air, intense sunlight—but ongoing nourishment from within. Deficiencies in the diet or physical imbalances and stress show up in the condition of the hair almost instantly.

Thus, diet is the primary factor in hair beauty; without this as the basis for the maintenance of hair health, the most determined external efforts are destined to fail. (Of course, diet alone will not ensure beautiful hair, easily damaged by improper handling and external aggressors like heat, harsh detergent shampoos, chemicals used in processing the hair, even careless brushing.)

In the Japanese diet, two foods in particular are eaten for maintaining or restoring the beauty of the hair: sesame seeds, especially the black variety, and sea plants, especially *kombu* and *nori*. Japanese babies, born with a feathery fluff of fine hair that wafts out in all directions like a dandelion flower gone to seed, are given *nori* to eat as soon as they are capable of consuming it in the conviction that the mineral-rich seaweed will give them strong, black, beautiful hair. Amazingly, it always works—though one suspects that natural tendencies too might play a large part in this development. Both sesame seeds and seaweed are eaten daily by the Japanese, and these are the commonly advised remedies when one is suffering from devitalized hair, graying hair, thin hair, or falling hair, or merely wishes to prevent such problems.

Other foods believed to contribute to the beauty of the hair are seafoods: shrimp, clams, sea cucumbers, sea urchins, fish roe, mackerel, sardines; the foods made from soybeans: tofu, *natto,* miso; lotus root, burdock root, carrots, cucumbers, apples, and perilla leaf. Brown rice, rice bran, azuki beans, and black soybeans are important as well. The Chinese wolfberry is eaten as a medicinal remedy for hair loss or graying.

Furikake, a mixture of such ingredients as *nori* flakes, fish roe, bits of dried sardine, and sesame seeds, is an excellent way to benefit from some of the Japanese hair-beauty foods. There are many different mixtures available commercially, but it is also a simple condiment to prepare at home with one's chosen ingredients. *Furikake* can be used as a highly nutritious and tasty seasoning to sprinkle over cooked grains, salads, vegetables, soups, and omelettes.

Many teas and broths presented in the facial care section also provide a good starting point for incorporating the Japanese ingredients.

The reader is reminded that where both skin and hair are concerned, the best results will be obtained by including the teas or foods in one's daily regimen over a period of months. If at the same time one conscientiously eliminates empty or harmful foods from the diet, both skin and hair will show improvements within a matter of weeks.

THE HAIR-CARE RITUAL

Daily or Less Frequently

Morning: Cleanse with a washing substance and massage.
Rinse (for as long as possible if the subsequent conditioning rinse is to be the final rinse).
Apply a conditioning rinse.
Rinse (if the conditioning rinse should be washed out) for as long as possible, finishing with a cold-water rinse.
Gently towel the hair dry.
Comb, applying an oil-in-water solution or a botanical mucilage for styling and protecting.
Apply a daytime treatment to the scalp if required.
Air dry or use a dryer at the lowest setting, stopping before the hair is completely dry.

Evening: Apply a nighttime treatment if required.

Weekly or As Needed

Morning
or
Evening: If a preshampoo treatment pack is used, apply it to the hair and have a soak in the bath or just relax, then proceed with the washing ritual as described above.
If a postshampoo treatment pack is used, first wash and rinse the hair, then apply the pack for the prescribed length of time. After rinsing, proceed with the usual sequence of steps, omitting the conditioning rinse if desired.

The teas described in chapter five may be incorporated into the daily regimen according to personal preference.

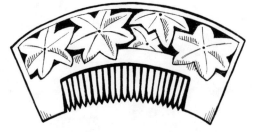

HAIR REGIMENS

A personal hair-care regimen may be designed by choosing à la carte from among the recipes in each section. Select a hair wash, a tea or rinse for conditioning, a treatment for occasional use, and if desired, a plain oil for day or night use or a special treatment oil for a specific need. Finally, choose a hair-beautifying tea to round out the program. Select recipes according to your hair type and immediate needs—the hair, like the skin, will vary in condition according to a wide range of factors such as diet, stress, season, and type of handling. As some of the ingredients—ginger and garlic, for example—are "hot" stimulants to the scalp, these may irritate sensitive skins, so they should be employed with care. Use small amounts at first, and gradually adjust the proportions if your scalp shows no adverse reactions. If irritation occurs, discontinue use of the substance. The scalp massage is an essential aspect of the Japanese approach to hair beauty; for a truly lovely, vibrant head of hair this step must be incorporated into the hair-care routine. The following regimens suggest appropriate programs for some common hair types and special needs.

Normal Hair
Rice Bran Shampoo
Camellia Water Rinse
Egg-Yolk Treatment Pack
Camellia Day/Night Oil
Cherry Bark Tea

Oily Hair
Violet Seaweed Shampoo
Brown Rice Vinegar Rinse
Honey Citron Rice Wine
Sesame Day/Night Oil
Simple Daikon Root Tea

Dry Hair
Sea Tangle Shampoo
Soybean Tea
Sesame Oil Treatment
Camellia Day/Night Oil
Seaweed Tea

Devitalized or Damaged Hair
Sea Tangle Shampoo
Soybean Tea
Garlic Rice Wine
Camellia Oil and Lemon Day/Night Treatment
Cherry Bark Tea

Frizzy, Flyaway, or Unmanageable Hair
Violet Seaweed Shampoo
Licorice Root Tea Rinse
Black Sugar Syrup Treatment Pack
Camellia Day/Night Oil
Seaweed Tea

Dandruff
Rice Bran Shampoo
Licorice Root Tea Rinse
Garlic Rice Wine
Sesame Day/Night Oil
Sweet Ginger *Kuzu* Tea

And for harmony with the seasons:

Spring
Pink Bean Powder and Olive Oil Shampoo
Camellia Water Rinse
Honey Citron Rice Wine
Camellia Day/Night Oil
Cherry Bark Tea

Summer
Whipped Egg-White Shampoo
Seaweed Tea Rinse
Egg-Yolk Treatment Pack
Camellia Oil and Lemon Day/Night Treatment
Seaweed Tea

Autumn
Rice Bran Shampoo
Soybean Tea
Sesame Oil With Ginger
Sesame Day/Night Oil
Sweet Ginger *Kuzu* Tea

Winter
Crushed Camellia Nut Shampoo
Soybean Tea
Black Sugar Syrup Treatment Pack
Sesame Day/Night Oil
Black Sesame *Kuzu* Tea

As an intensive short-term beauty cure for the hair, this regimen may be followed for three weeks or so:

The Potent Hair-Beauty Cure
Violet Seaweed Shampoo
Seaweed Tea Rinse
Garlic Rice Wine
Sesame Oil with Ginger Day/Night Treatment
Seaweed Tea

The Japanese Comb

The Japanese comb goes way back, back to the time when the gods and goddesses were creating the mountains and rivers and valleys and hot springs of Japan. The comb of a goddess could be used to make a waterfall or erect a small mountain, rather a useful object in the task of arranging the world.

It stands to reason that if a woman's hair is her most alluring adornment, her most precious treasure, that if beautiful hair is so powerfully enchanting that a woman can capture a man's love with beautiful hair alone, then the comb is a valuable item indeed. The hair invites love with the comb's help.

Symbolic of magic, beauty, and love, a Japanese comb must be accorded the appropriate care and respect. To break a comb is a bad omen. To give a comb as a gift suggests the final *sayonara*. A comb received from one's lover is thrown away when the romance ends. (Though one has to wonder about the motives of the lover who presents the comb in the first place. This has always puzzled me.)

The magical pitfalls of the Japanese comb notwithstanding, the utensil itself is a remarkable tool for beauty. The traditional wisdom has it that a brush should never be used on the hair, as this will cause breakage and splitting. The traditional boxwood comb, *tsuge no kushi,* is made with thick, closely spaced teeth with blunted tips. Used for grooming the hair, the comb simultaneously delivers a stimulating massage to the scalp, provided one combs with it properly, applying the comb directly to the scalp and not only to the hair. This daily stimulation, in combination with frequent scalp massage, is believed to be valuable in preventing hair loss and improving the circulation of the scalp, thus supplying an increase of nutrients to the hair follicles. This in turn encourages the healthy growth of the hair and improves tone and color, resulting in hair that has a rich texture and a naturally silky shine.

A wooden comb should not be washed in soapy water, but should be brushed with a comb brush and cleaned and protected by the occasional application of camellia oil.

Hairdressing Oils

For centuries women (and men) in Japan have been taming and sculpting their hair with these oils.

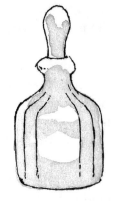

Actions:

Nourishes
Moisturizes
Gives luster

Indications:

All hair types
Use as needed

Ingredients:

Camellia nut oil, or sesame oil, or castor oil, or walnut oil

Directions for Use:

An oil may be applied directly to the hair for styling and conditioning, but this method leaves the hair rather oiled, which may be desirable for some hairstyles and hair types, but not for others. An alternative method is to add a drop or two of oil to warm water in a basin, then dip fingers or comb into the water to apply to hair and style.

Simple Flower-Dew Oil

Actions:

Heals
Purifies
Moisturizes
Gives luster

Indications:

All skin and hair types
Use as needed

Ingredients:

Chopped sandalwood
Cloves
Sesame Oil

Preparation:

Fill a lidded jar with sandalwood and cloves, then add sesame oil to cover. Seal the jar tightly and let it sit for 10 days, shaking it occasionally. The mixture may be strained, returning the oil to the jar with a new batch of sandalwood and cloves, to repeat the process. Filter through silk, and store in a sealed bottle.

Directions for Use:

Apply the oil to skin and hair. For application to the hair, the oil may be applied in tiny amounts as is (with oily results), or by adding a drop or two to a basin of warm water, into which a comb is dipped for styling.

The designation hananotsuyu *"flower-dew" oil, started out as a brand name for a remarkable scented medicinal oil developed in the mid-1600s by a hunchback called Kizaemon. The oil, which contained aromatic and curative essential oils, was said to eliminate pimples and give a luster to the complexion when used on the face. As women were apt to apply the same oils or pomades to their hair as they used on their faces,* hananotsuyu *gradually became known as a hair oil, too.*

123

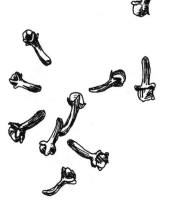

PART THREE

THE BEAUTY OF THE BODY

THE BEAUTY OF THE BODY

The heart and soul of the Japanese way of beauty is the bath. The bath is where everything comes together: the rituals of face, hair, and body care; cleansing; simple sensual pleasure; renewal of the spirit; mental relaxation; even the harmony between self and others. The ceremony of bathing is for the Japanese a daily rite, a return to the source, a time of delicious, languorous immersion in the hot, all-healing waters. In the bath, one peacefully surrenders to spiritual-terrestrial bliss, to emerge newly purified once again.

Blessed with an abundance of hot water from the earth, Japan is a land of 20,000 thermal springs, a land where white monkeys soak in steaming mountain pools amid towering snowdrifts, where entire villages exist because of the medicinal waters bubbling up from some volcanic source, where illnesses of all kinds are treated by bathing. The centering, curative, beautifying, spirit-soothing effects are acknowledged by all.

The highly developed ritual that is bathing in Japan almost certainly originated with ancient Shinto, which worshipped the sacred in nature and which placed a primary emphasis on purification. To immerse oneself in a hot-spring bath was thus an act of religious cleansing, and also a time to contemplate the elemental forces of nature, aided in this by the meditative state induced by the bath.

Sitting naked in a hot mineral bath, clouds of steam wafting and billowing from the water, surrounded by big gleaming rocks, a misty forest of all pines, the silence of snow, one experiences an intimate human compatibility with nature, a magnificently simple harmony with the elements. The warm camaraderie between fellow bathers, the impression of timelessness that comes with living fully in the here and now, the voluptuous sense of doing nothing, submitting one's being to the combined powers of water and heat—such a bath envelops body, mind, and spirit in a deep and luxurious relaxation.

When one has bathed in such a Japanese hot spring, soaked chin-deep in a mountain pool with friends or family until the ordinary world has melted away like a dream, one understands the presence of the large communal public bath in every neighborhood, the roomy, deep, soaking tub in every Japanese home, the long, hot soak every evening, the family-shared bathtime. The Japanese bath is a lesson learned from nature.

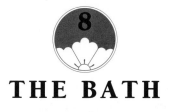

THE BATH

*I*took my first Japanese bath in Kyoto, in a small and ascetically beautiful traditional inn. I was ten or eleven years old, and that bath seemed to me like something out of a fairy tale or a dream. The square wooden tub, made of smooth, unfinished Japanese cypress, was very big and very deep. The hot water that filled it reached exactly to the rim, and floating upon the steaming surface were a few slices of yellow citron, *yuzu.* Soaking in the bath, I could gaze out upon the *ryokan* garden: green moss, dewy gray rocks, a flowering tree. The surroundings were peaceful, elegant, both simple and luxurious. Colors were muted, the light was the natural soft light from the garden outside, the only sounds were water sounds. Surfaces were wetly gleaming stone and tile, with blond wood and bamboo ladles, buckets, bathstool, floor. The bath was pure enchantment.

The evening bath is a daily ritual in Japan. Every home is equipped with a bathing room designed for presoak washing, a spacious area in which are placed bathstools and basins, dippers and sponges, with a hand-held shower or faucet to provide running water. The bathtub is entered only after one is thoroughly washed and rinsed.

While bathwater may be simply plain, clear hot water, there is a long tradition in Japan of adding some natural substance to the bath for medicinal, beautifying, aromatic, body-warming, invigorating, purifying, symbolic, or magical purposes. Baths may contain flowers such as iris, rose, chrysanthemum; leaves such as daikon, carrot, cherry, peach; fruits such as citron, tangerine, orange; roots such as lotus, ginger, iris; rice products such as *sake,* vinegar, rice bran; a variety of seaweeds. While the purist will employ the raw material, harvesting the leaves, roots, and flowers herself for drying and adding to the bath, many Japanese companies now offer prepared bath herbs and salts, which present all the traditional substances in handy packet form.

One bathes to purify oneself but also to soothe and relax body and mind, to recharge the being, to release tensions, to drift while the being is revitalized. The home bath, taken in solitude, is a time for centering, rebalancing, for recovering a sense of well-being. The bath is a pleasant and sensual way to achieve a state of deep mental relaxation. The bath taken with friends and family is a time for idle conversation, a sharing of warmth and enjoyment, for scrubbing backs, and simply for being together.

To increase circulation benefits, aid in elimination, and to prevent dehydration and dizziness, a tea made from soy sauce and ginger may be drunk before bathing. One teaspoonful of freshly grated and squeezed ginger root juice is added to double the amount of soy sauce; to this is added some *bancha* tea. An optional addition is a pitted, mashed *umeboshi*—though the taste will be sour, stimulation of the circulation and elimination functions will be increased. Simple water or juice taken prebath will provide protection against dehydration.

Salt added to the bathwater will help to prevent the dizziness and extreme fatigue sometimes caused by hot-water bathing; this is especially useful for a bather who is weak or elderly (though in general, such persons should avoid temperature extremes). The best time to bathe is when the stomach is empty, but not when very hungry. Wait for several hours after eating, or bathe before having a meal.

A bath taken in the morning should be a tonic bath, one which will encourage the elimination of toxins and stimulate the organism. The temperature for a tonic, invigorating bath is around 96.8 degrees Fahrenheit (36 degrees centigrade) and the duration should be around ten minutes. The tonic bath will relieve physical fatigue at whatever time it is taken.

An evening bath is generally a relaxing bath, taken for fifteen to twenty minutes at a temperature of 98.6 degrees Fahrenheit (37 degrees centigrade) to 102 degrees Fahrenheit (39 degrees centigrade), though some prefer a higher temperature. This bath relieves nervous tension, mental fatigue, and stress, encouraging an easy and deep sleep.

The bath of 104 degrees Fahrenheit (40 degrees centigrade) to 107 degrees Fahrenheit (42 degrees centigrade) is ideal for muscle aches and pains and after physical exertion. This bath should be taken for a short time. While one often hears that very hot baths will cause sagging and wrinkling of the skin, recent evidence suggests otherwise. Judging by the general Japanese population's skin condition—remarkably smooth and firm, lacking in sags, wrinkles, and cellulite— I am inclined to agree with the new findings. The daily Japanese bath is commonly between 104 degrees and 107 degrees Fahrenheit. Certainly, the very young, the very old, and anyone in a weak or convalescing condition, or anyone with hypertension, poor circulation, heart conditions or blood pressure problems should stick to less fiery temperatures.

After a hot bath, a cold-water shower will tone the skin and increase resistance to colds and infections. In the Japanese way of bathing, this step, though not regularly practiced by everyone, is commonly advised as one of the best ways of strengthening the body.

After a toxin-eliminating bath, a rest period during which one reclines, wrapped snugly in an absorbent robe and a blanket, for a period of time equivalent to the time spent soaking, will allow for maximum benefits. The rest period is followed by a warm-water scrub, a cool shower, and the application of an oil, emollient, or plant water.

One generally feels rather thirsty after emerging from a hot bath, and it is important to replenish the body's fluids by drinking water or tea postbath.

For those who are unaccustomed to long hot bath-soaks, these simple rules should be observed: Prior to immersion, douse the body and head repeatedly with water from the bath. Five to ten minutes of such dousing—or showering—will enable the body to adjust to the heat more easily. Don't expect to develop hot-bath tolerance overnight; the best approach is to train oneself gradually over a period of time, going from warm to warmer to hot temperatures and increasing soaking periods little by little. Finally, it is unwise to stand up suddenly when emerging from a hot bath—dizziness and even fainting are common dangers.

While the true Japanese bath experience can only be had in a room with all the right amenities—an area for out-of-tub washing and showering, a deep and roomy soaking tub, a peaceful view of nature to inspire bathtime contemplation and serene reverie—one may approximate the ritual even in a typical Western-style bathing room. This may be done by showering and washing first, thoroughly rinsing both self and bathtub, then filling the tub for a soak. The room should be warmed ahead of time to avoid chilling.

Lowered lights, a whiff of some subtle plum blossom or pine incense, perhaps the faintly heard plucking of a *koto* in the background, or an ambiance tape all help to induce serenity.

The steps in the Japanese bath:

- Prepare bath by filling with water and adding bath ingredient(s), either directly into the water or tied into a cloth bag to float. (A good method of infusing plant ingredients is to tie the bag to the faucet, filling the bath with hot water only for an initial ten to fifteen minutes, then adding cool water to achieve the appropriate temperature.)
- Drink water, juice, or tea.
- Wash and scrub the body thoroughly (using a shower or faucet separate from the soaking tub).
- Rinse well.
- Apply treatment packs to the face and hair if desired.
- Soak. Relax. Let the mind drift.
- Scrub and soak alternately, if desired.
- After a final scrubbing and a thorough rinse, shower with cool or cold water.
- Towel dry and apply an oil, emollient, or plant water.

Rice Bran Bath

In the Japanese tradition, this is the bath of baths. Versions of the rice bran bath have been taken for centuries in this land of bath connoisseurs. It may be that this is *The Perfect Bath*, as simple as that. It cleanses splendidly, heals, nourishes, moisturizes, and beautifies. It is everything one might want in a bath, and more.

130

Actions:

Cleanses
Nourishes
Stimulates skin metabolism
Heals
Softens
Moisturizes
Soothes irritations, rashes, sunburn

Indications:

All skin types
Bathe as frequently as desired

Ingredients:

3½ pounds (1½ kilos) fresh rice bran
Water

Preparation:

Fasten the rice bran securely in a muslin bag, then place it in a nonmetal pot containing five times as much water as bran. Boil the water for 15 minutes, then add the bran bag and liquid to a tepid bath.

Directions for Bathing:

Soak for 20 to 30 minutes. Do not rinse.

Skin-Like-a-Gleaming-Jewel Rice Wine Bath

Actions:

Regenerates
Eases fatigue and sore muscles
Invigorates
Eliminates toxins
Smooths skin
Stimulates circulation
Warms
Encourages perspiration

Indications:

All skin types
Weekly

Ingredients:

2 quarts (2 liters) or so of rice wine

Preparation:

Fill the bathtub with hot water; when it is ready, add 1 to 2 liters of *sake*.

Directions for Use:

It is best to soak for at least 30 minutes in the rice wine bath. Although the body is thoroughly washed and scrubbed prior to bathing, the rice wine so efficiently encourages the elimination of toxins that by the end of the soak the bathwater will be very visibly dirty.

The rice wine bath is three thousand years old. Though it has healing properties— the elimination of toxins, the stimulation of circulation, the easing of sore muscles—it is most legendary for its enhancement of beauty. Skin is so smoothed and softened by the sakeburo *that the bath sake sold in Japan is called* tama no hada sake, *"skin-like-a-gleaming-jewel-sake." Any rice wine will do for this bath.*

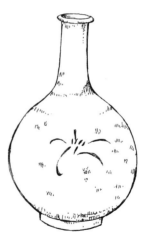

Bath of Rice Vinegar

This summer bath is taken for its enriching supply of amino acids and its ability to decrease the quantity of lactic acid in the blood, often caused by strenuous exercise. The skin is balanced, toned, and softened by this refreshing, sweetly sour bath.

Actions:

Neutralizes lactic acid
Cleanses
Refreshes
Relieves fatigue and sore or stiff muscles
Lightens
Stimulates circulation

Indications:

All skin types
Bathe as frequently as desired

Ingredients:

2 cups (480 ml) brown rice vinegar

Preparation:

Add vinegar to a tepid bath.

Directions for Bathing:

Soak for 15 to 20 minutes; rinsing is not necessary.

Bath of Ginseng Root

Actions:

Tones
Smooths
Softens
Refines

Indications:

All skin types
Recommended for rough or dry skin
Bathe as frequently as desired

Ingredients:

Several pieces of ginseng root
4¼ cups (1 liter) pure spring water

Preparation:

Place ginseng and cold water in a covered nonmetal pan and bring to a boil, then reduce the flame and simmer until the volume is reduced to 25 percent of the original amount. Steep at room temperature, still covered, until cool.

Add water and roots to a hot bath.

Directions for Bathing:

Soak for 20 to 30 minutes.

Ginseng, like many other tonic herbs used internally, is useful also as an external treatment. In the bath, ginseng is said to tone and refine the skin, making it sleek, soft, and truly silky.

133

Ginger Bath

The powers of the pungent ginger root are many: used in a bath, it is stimulating, invigorating, warming, relaxing, curative, purifying, soothing, beautifying, and will help to prevent or cure a cold. A ginger bath will relieve chapped skin, frostbite, fatigue, overexercised or stiff muscles, and can even make one feel more lighthearted, or so they say.

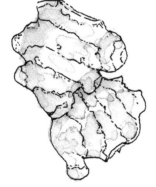

Actions:

Stimulates
Eliminates toxins
Relieves muscle pain
Causes sweating
Relaxes tension
Warms
Soothes

Indications:

Not recommended for sensitive skin
Bathe weekly (more frequent ginger baths may cause adverse reactions)

Ingredients:

2 or 3 large ginger roots

Preparation:

Grate the ginger, squeeze it through a cloth to obtain juice, and add the juice to a hot bath.

Directions for Bathing:

Soak long enough to induce sweating. Rinse.

(Any irritation or burning sensations are a sign that less ginger should be used. If such symptoms are severe, it is wise to forego future baths of ginger.)

Winter Garlic Bath

Actions:

Warms
Stimulates circulation
Improves metabolism
Aids relaxation
Induces sleep
Soothes aches and pains

Indications:

Not recommended for those with sensitive skin
Bathe as frequently as desired

Ingredients:

Cloves of fresh garlic

Preparation:

Peel garlic cloves and add as many as you like
to a hot bath.

Directions for Bathing:

Soak. This bath is very good for combating
insomnia; because it is warming and deeply
relaxing, it is the perfect bath for a cold winter's
night, just before bedtime.

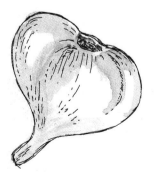

Most of my Japanese friends consider the garlic bath rather eccentric, even perverse. Who would willingly immerse her delicate feminine self in a whole bathful of garlic aroma? But the garlic bath is in fact an ancient traditional bath with extraordinary potency as a tonic for health and beauty.

These days in Japan one can buy powdered odorless garlic bath salts, but purists say that there's nothing like the real thing. As with the other garlic treatments, the garlic bath has an almost magical reputation as a strengthener, purifier and protector, being effective against neuralgia, lumbago, rheumatism, stiff muscles, insomnia, and weakness, as well as being of benefit to bruises, heat rash, eczema, and frostbite, constipation, menstrual problems, low blood pressure, and colds.

Fennel Stalk Bath

Have a sweet-scented fennel bath to make your skin more beautiful, smooth, soft, pure, calm, clean, soothed, refreshed, and stimulated. Also, the bath is warming.

Actions:

Warms
Stimulates
Soothes

Indications:

All skin types
Bathe as frequently as desired

Ingredients:

Fresh fennel stalks

Preparation:

Chop some fresh whole fennel stalks, place in a gauze square and fasten.

Add the bag to a hot bath.

Directions for Bathing:

Soak.

136

New Year's Day Pine Bath

Actions:

Purifies
Stimulates circulation
Invigorates
Eases stiffness, aches, neuralgia, rheumatism
Refreshes
Tones

Indications:

All skin types
Bathe as frequently as desired

Ingredients:

Fresh pine needles

Preparation:

Pine needles may be used fresh or dried. To dry, suspend branches in a shady spot for a week or so, then store wrapped in paper in a cool, dry location.

Wrap fresh or dried pine needles in a gauze square and tie securely. Place in a hot bath.

Directions for Bathing:

Soak for 20 to 30 minutes for deep relaxation and regeneration.

Japanese fairy tales are full of enchanted pine trees, pine-tree princesses and princes, talking pine trees, and pine-tree-dwelling spirits. Even the more ordinary pine trees of Japan, the tall old pines in mountain forests, the twisted, dancing pines of the islands at Matsushima, the sculpted pines inhabiting every garden—even these pine trees seem surrounded by a magically vital atmosphere. Perhaps it is because they are trees beloved by an entire nation. A spirit-renewing bath of evergreen pine is auspicious for the New Year.

137

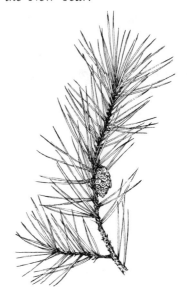

Sweet Flag Bath, in Honor of Boy Children

The sword-like leaves of the sweet-smelling medicinal sweet flag are added to baths all over Japan on Boys' Day, May 5. The plant has been used for centuries to guard against evil; its use in the bath is said to purify both mind and body, ensuring continuing health and strength for all, but especially the boy children honored on this day.

Sweet flag water, or shobu-yu, is said to cure skin infections, help sprains to heal, eliminate fatigue, prevent against illness, improve general health, and smooth and soften the skin in the bargain. Though imperative for Boys' Day, the sweet flag bath may be taken any time the lavender-flowering shobu is in bloom.

Actions:

Improves circulation
Warms
Prevents colds
Strengthens

Indications:

All skin types
Bathe as frequently as desired

Ingredients:

Fresh leaves of sweet flag (a plant very similar to the iris)

Preparation:

Tie a generous bundle of sweet flag leaves with cord. (The roots are beneficial as well and should not be removed, just washed to eliminate dirt.) The leaf bundle is added to the hot bathwater.

Directions for Bathing:

Relax and soak in the fragrant water while it works its magic. Do not rinse.

Yellow Chrysanthemum Bath

Actions:

Warms
Rejuvenates
Heals cuts and scratches
Reduces scarring
Destroys bacteria
Tones skin

Indications:

Any skin type
Bathe as frequently as desired

Ingredients:

Edible yellow chrysanthemums

Preparation:

Float chrysanthemum flowers in a hot bath.

Directions for Bathing:

Soak; do not rinse.

The noble chrysanthemum of October is the flower of longevity and youth. The chrysanthemum of Japan is honored with its own festival, is cultivated with exquisite care in home gardens, is used as a dainty edible garnish for elegant meals, and is used medicinally to destroy germs. It is also found adorning the evening bath, where it is used not only for warming, but also, if there is truth in the legend, to keep the ravages of age at bay. Yellow chrysanthemum makes a healing, warming, youth-giving bath for the crisp evenings of early autumn.

139

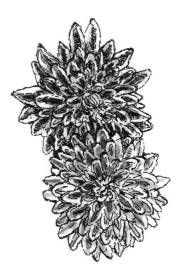

Stimulating Mustard Bath

This is a hot bath, in all senses of the word. A mustard bath is warming and stimulating, said to improve the circulation, speed up the metabolism, relieve muscle aches and pains, and even act as an aphrodisiac. The bath also helps to relieve fatigue, lassitude, chills, and despondency.

Actions:

Stimulates
Relieves muscle pain

Indications:

Not recommended for sensitive or irritated skin
Bathe weekly or as needed

Ingredients:

½ cup (120 cc) powdered mustard

Preparation:

Mix mustard powder with some cold water, then add to a tepid bath.

Directions for Bathing:

Soak for 10 or 15 minutes, then rinse. If any irritation is experienced, stop bathing immediately and rinse well. Children should not take this bath.

Bath of Spring Rose Petals

Actions:

Soothes
Heals
Softens
Perfumes and deodorizes
Calms
Astringes

Indications:

All skin types
Recommended for irritated skin, sensitive skin,
  and dry skin
Bathe as frequently as desired

Ingredients:

Fresh-picked rose petals

Preparation:

Sprinkle a few handfuls of rose petals in a tepid
bath.

Directions for Bathing:

Soak.

The sweet scent of rose perfumes this gently healing bath. The rose bath will soften and soothe the skin, making it as velvety to the touch as the flower petal itself. A romantic bath for a cool evening in late spring.

Tangerine Bath

The sweet tangerines of winter offer a favorite Japanese warming bath. Whether dried peels or the whole fruits are set to float like mystical globes of orange in the hot water, the bath is aromatic, delightful, and spirit-soothing.

142

Actions:

Stimulates circulation
Smoothes skin
Nourishes
Moisturizes
Perfumes

Indications:

All skin types
Recommended for poor circulation, chapped skin
Bathe as frequently as desired

Ingredients:

Tangerine or mandarin orange peels, or the
    whole fresh fruits

Preparation:

Spread the peels to dry in a shady location. When they are thoroughly dried, after a week or ten days, store them in a sealed, moisture-free container. The peels will keep indefinitely.

For the bath, break the dried peels into small bits, then tie into a piece of gauze and fasten with a cord.

Directions for Bathing:

Place the bag or 4 or 5 whole tangerines in a hot bath, then soak.

December Citron Bath

Actions:

Warms
Improves circulation
Moisturizes
Relieves aches and tension, neuralgia, lumbago
Softens rough skin
Perfumes and deodorizes
Astringes

Indications:

All skin types
Recommended for chapped skin, poor
    circulation, tension
Bathe as frequently as desired

Ingredients:

Citron peels, or the whole fresh fruits (lemons
    may be substituted)

Preparation:

Prepare the peels as for the Tangerine Bath.

If whole fruits are used, they may be sliced into
rounds.

Directions for Bathing:

Place the bag of peels, a few whole fruits, or
round slices in the hot bath, then soak.

The yuzu, or citron, is possessed of an enchanting, feminine fragrance. When I smelled its perfume the first time, I had the mysterious sensation of encountering something perfectly surprising, unknown, and at the same time inexplicably familiar. The lemon could substitute for the sour yellow citron, but for its ineffable fragrance. Japanese tradition holds that a yuzu-yu bath taken on the day of the Winter Solstice will guard against colds all winter; aromatherapists say yuzu makes one optimistic.

143

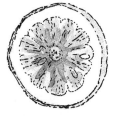

Hot Ocean Bath

In this volcanically active land, located in heady proximity to the Ring of Fire linking various Pacific hot spots, the ocean is nevertheless reassuringly cold—frigid, in fact. There are hot springs that are salty and very hot, and perhaps this bath resembles such salt springs more than it does the Sea of Japan. But it is sea salt that makes this bath, and it brings with it all the rich benefits of seawater.

Actions:

Relaxes
Tones and tightens skin
Invigorates
Smooths

Indications:

All skin types
Recommended for the elderly and the weak
Bathe as frequently as desired

Ingredients:

4 cups (900 cc) coarse sea salt

Preparation:

Add salt to a bath which is a little below body temperature, around 97° F (36° C). Powdered seaweed may be added if desired.

Directions for Bathing:

Soak for 15 minutes, adding some hot water if the temperature is uncomfortable. Rinse after bathing.

The Japanese Bathtub

The traditional Japanese bathtub is the *hinokiburo*, fashioned from fragrant Japanese cypress. Pale blond in color, it is smooth and silky to the touch, its beautiful grain and soft texture kept in a natural unfinished state, polished by fine sanding to a satiny sheen. The wood of *hinoki* lends itself perfectly to use in the bathtub, with its high resistance to moisture, its ability to eliminate odors, and its antibacterial properties. Further, this wood's natural oils are said to reduce inflammations and induce calm and, due to the particularly penetrative nature of the substance, to impart these benefits to the *hinokiburo* bather. The same durable wood is used for sushi-shop chopping boards; its sterilizing properties and its softness— the ultra-sharp fish-slicing knives are not dulled or damaged by the wood—make it indispensable. The extract of *hinoki* is a fundamental ingredient in many Japanese skin-care and cosmetics products; there is even a fresh-scented, anti-inflammatory toothpaste made from it.

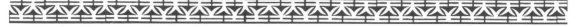

Tonic Seaweed Bath

The ocean-scented seaweed bath is the ultimate revitalizing soak. Full of vitamins and minerals, it is both curative and beautifying. To take this bath properly, allowing for the maximum elimination of toxins, the prolonged penetration of active substances, and the most effective boost to circulation, metabolism, and other body functions, it must be followed by a wrapped-up rest period equivalent in length to the time spent bathing.

146

Actions:

Regenerates

Deep-cleanses

Tones

Stimulates cell activity
and circulation

Soothes sunburn

Eliminates toxins

Nourishes

Indications:

All skin types

Recommended for fatigue, stress, devitalized skin

Bathe weekly

Ingredients:

Any edible seaweeds: *kombu, wakame, funori* in
    leaf or powder form

Preparation:

Dried seaweed must be soaked for 20 minutes in tepid water before use—this may be done directly in the bath—and salted seaweed must be rinsed.

Leaf seaweed may be tied into a piece of gauze and secured with a cord, or it may be added to the bath as is. Powdered seaweed may be sprinkled directly into the water.

Directions for Bathing:

Soak in water that is tepid to hot (100° F [38° C] to 107° F [42° C]) for 20 minutes.

Upon emerging from the bath immediately wrap up snugly in a thick robe, then lie down for a rest under a quilt or blanket, with feet and head raised slightly on pillows. After resting like this for 20 minutes or more, then shower and scrub the body.

Alkaline Bath

Actions:

Softens
Stimulates circulation
Warms
Relaxes
Soothes sore muscles
Invigorates
Eliminates toxins

Indications:

All skin types
Bathe as frequently as desired

Ingredients:

3 tablespoons (45 cc) baking soda

Preparation:

Add baking soda to a hot bath.

Directions for Bathing:

Soak; do not rinse.

This is a bath inspired by the hot-spring tradition. Simple baking soda used in the bath will soften the skin while it relieves fatigue, tension, aches, and pains.

THE FOOTBATH

The footbath is a curative bath, a folk remedy known to wise grandmothers all over Japan. Advised for cases of insomnia, a cold, poor circulation, or simple winter chills, there are a number of variations. One easy footbath is to pour a bucketful of rather hot water over the ankles and feet after soaking in the bath. The water should be hotter than that used for soaking. The saltwater footbath is another method: a bit of sea salt is added to very hot water in a footbath tub, in which the feet are placed for ten minutes or so while one sits peacefully in a chair. The water should be kept as hot as possible by adding hotter water every now and then. The final footbath variation involves two footbath tubs, one filled with hot water (kept hot as described above), and the other filled with cold water. Sitting in a chair, one sits with the feet in the hot bath for thirty to sixty seconds, then places them in the cold bath for an equal amount of time. This back-and-forth ritual is repeated for about fifteen minutes, until the body feels warm through and through. (For a cold, drink a cup of *bancha* tea with an *umeboshi* in it during your footbath.) Any of the footbath variations is meant to be taken just before retiring for the night. For extra stimulation and warming, prepare the Mustard Bath, the Chrysanthemum Bath, or the Ginger Bath (using lesser amounts of the ingredients) as a footbath.

THE HIPBATH

Another localized bath technique, known in the West as the sitz bath, is the hipbath, used in Japan as a stimulating, warming, curative bath, particularly for women. The bath is prepared by filling a washtub with rather hot water, then sitting in the water so that only the derrière, hips, and waist area are immersed. The rest of the body should be covered. The bath is taken for a period of twenty to thirty minutes, adding hotter water when it begins to cool. The hipbath is often advised in order to strengthen and balance the constitution, improve the functioning of reproductive and eliminatory systems, and to increase a woman's interest in lovemaking. It is said in Japan that the hipbath is a powerful method of toning and healing the entire system. To intensify curative properties, the Ginger Bath (see page 134) may be used as a hipbath.

THE BODY-POLISHING
BATH SCRUB

For skin that is pearly, lustrous, and smooth, skin as soft and translucent as a baby's, for a body contour that is toned, streamlined, and taut (without bumps, bulges, sags, and cellulite), the secret is a simple one: scrub. The Japanese bath is a finely developed art, composed of two complementary rituals—the thorough body scrub and the prolonged deep-relaxation soak.

Any visitor to a Japanese public bath or hot-spring spa will see the scrub-and-soak process vividly enacted. A bather seats herself upon her bathstool, sets up her personal array of sponges, brushes, mitts, pumice stones, soaps, shampoos, and potions, fills her small basin with water from one of the many faucets provided, and begins her preliminary cleansing scrub. This scrub is prolonged and energetic, a very active, very attentive cleansing of the body from head to toe. Once scrubbed and rinsed, the bather enters the bath for her initial soaking period, during which time she rests in a state of passive contemplation while the hot water melts away all tension.

When this first soak is over, the bather goes again to her washing-stool, where she will once again scrub. This time, she is sure to become even cleaner, for the hot water and steam have opened her pores and begun to stimulate the elimination of toxins through the skin. She may follow up the scrub this time with an icy shower or a few cold dousings with bucket or basin. Again, the bather, now pink and rosy, settles into the hot bath for more soaking. And again, she will emerge to scrub, and again immerse to soak. The process will continue for as long as she can devote to it—usually no less than thirty minutes, often for more than an hour.

The scrubbing process serves several purposes. Most obvious are cleansing and exfoliating—the complete removal of dirt, toxins, and the dead, dull outer layer of skin cells. The scrubbing of the body is also a stimulating massage, acting to revitalize the skin circulation and metabolism, bringing blood and nutrients to the surface, causing skin to glow with lively health and vitality. Vigorous scrubbing is also said to be an excellent method of pressure-point stimulation.

In comparison with the Japanese scrubbing ritual, the standard Western body-wash—a superficial and perfunctory once-over with soap—seems indeed rudimentary. The Japanese have long grasped the primary importance of both external and internal cleanliness. The skin is an organ of elimination, discharging more than a pound of waste daily through its pores. What happens, not only to the skin, but to less visible parts of the body when such waste is not actively removed?

During years of communal bathing in Japan, I have never seen a single woman with cellulite. Is the body-scrub tradition a factor in this? The Japanese believe that the skin must be stimulated and "worked" in order to discourage the formation of fat deposits, dead, sagging areas, and stiffness caused by the accumulation of tension. The internal counterpart to the cleansing, enlivening scrub is a diet which includes many foods consumed entirely for their ability to purify, strengthen, and help the body to eliminate toxins.

The Japanese bath is a social ritual, and mutual back-scrubbing is a beloved part of the bath taken with friends or family. In every Japanese home, it is the custom for even tiny children to scrub their parents' backs, thus learning at the impressionable age of two or three that bathtime scrubbing is an enjoyable and essential element of the daily routine.

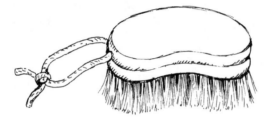

To benefit circulation, improve resistance to colds and infections, to soften, smooth, and revitalize the skin, to refine the silhouette, and to make the body less vulnerable to chilly temperatures, the entire body should be scrubbed on a daily basis, even if only for five minutes. Every few days, time should be set aside for a longer session, with alternated scrubbing and soaking.

Scrubbing is always practiced with the utmost respect for the skin. The skin is stimulated but not abraded or irritated, and appropriately textured scrubbing tools are utilized for the various surfaces of the body. The beginning body-scrubber is advised to start out with caution and delicacy; the skin will gradually become stronger, until an enthusiastic and vigorous rubdown will be possible. In Japan, skin-scrubbing is thought of as endurance training for the skin, a disciplining process whereby the skin grows healthier, tougher, more resilient.

Most of the body, with the exception of the face, may be scrubbed with a rather stiff brush, mitt, or loofah, adjusting the pressure according to the tenderness of each area. Breasts, inner thighs, and inner arms require a gentle touch. For feet, knees, and elbows, a very stiff brush or pumice stone may be employed. On the face and neck areas, a soft facial brush, cleansing bag, or sea sponge may be used.

The steps in the Japanese body-scrub

- For a dry friction scrub, apply no water or cleansing ingredient to the skin or scrubber. Brush as described, from extremities toward the heart. (This dry scrub may precede a wet scrub.) Rinse.
- For a wet scrub, moisten the body with warm water.
- If you are using a bag filled with a cleansing ingredient, soak the bag in warm water. If using a sponge, brush, mitt, or towel, apply a cleansing ingredient to the moistened scrubber.
- Scrub as directed, with soft and gentle strokes if your skin is not adapted to scrubbing. If this scrub is the first of several during the bathing session, you need not be terribly thorough. If it is the only scrub, spend at least five minutes on comprehensive scrubbing. Rinse.
- Soak in rather hot water for a minimum of five minutes.
- The next scrub should be more thorough than the first. Rinse.
- Soak again.
- Scrub. (The number of scrubs varies from bather to bather; usually there is a minimum of two per long session, a maximum of four or five.) Rinse.
- The last scrub is followed by a cold-water rinse.
- Dry gently, apply moisturizer, and relax.

While the modern-day bather may choose from a variety of soaps, body shampoos, and cleansing creams, traditionally the body was scrubbed with rice bran, a mixture of rice bran and azuki bean powder, crushed camellia nuts, or occasionally seaweed. A body-scrubbing bag, somewhat larger than that used for the face, was fashioned out of fine cotton or silk, filled with the cleansing ingredients, soaked before washing, then used to thoroughly scrub and massage every part of the body.

The scrubbing ritual is most commonly practiced wet, but some bathers prefer to begin the process with a dry friction scrub. This is very invigorating, and one can actually see the dead skin flying off!

Whatever scrubbing method is employed, the basic technique is always the same. Use your brush, bag, towel, or sponge in a careful circular motion, starting at the extremities and moving toward the heart area. Beginning at the feet, spiral up the legs, then move to the hands and up the arms, and finally to the torso, front and back, always directing the strokes toward the heart. Circle gently around the breasts and abdomen, and if using a towel or long sponge or bag, wash the back with long diagonal strokes. Avoid moles, warts, blemishes, and varicose veins.

The Japanese bathing room, designed as it is for outside-the-tub washing and scrubbing—usually with a flexible shower and faucets, an area with stools and basins for sit-down cleansing, and a big, deep tub that may be filled beforehand—obviously provides the best physical arrangement for the scrub-soak ritual. Dirt and soap are strangers to the bathwater, which must remain pure for soaking. To practice this ritual in a standard Western bath is more difficult. Perhaps the closest one can come to it is first performing a dry friction scrub, followed by a very thorough shower-scrub, a complete rinsing of the body and bathtub, and then filling the tub for a soak. After a lengthy soak, follow up with a final shower-scrub, a good rinsing, and then a cold shower for a minute or two.

(How primitive it seems to bathe Western-style! To luxuriate in a tub full of soapy, dirty water is an incongruous custom, showing an eminent lack of common sense. The Japanese bathing system is much more logical and civilized, and certainly more aesthetically appealing.)

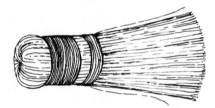

SKIN-SCRUBBING AND POLISHING TOOLS

Japan has always been known for its elegantly designed, sublimely simple functional tools and utensils for everyday needs. Superbly crafted in natural materials, such tools impart to the most humble task a sense of grace and quiet ritual.

From earliest times, the Japanese bath has been both a ceremony of purification and a practical necessity, and the objects used in bathing are among the most beautiful of Japanese crafts. Traditional bathtubs, stools, ladles, scoops, and buckets made of sweet-smelling cypress combine purity of line with the sensual warmth of smooth, unfinished wood.

A visit to a Japanese bath-goods store will reveal the astonishing array of scrubbing tools available to the bather: natural-bristle body brushes of every shape and size, delicate complexion brushes, sea sponges large and petite, hemp friction straps and mitts, silk mitts and bags, cotton bags and straps, abrasive sponges and wash towels, turtle-shaped *tawashi* brushes, pumice stones, devil's tongue root sponges, milk sponges and towels, and loofah sponges three feet long.

There are tools with clever curved handles for reaching remote regions of the back, tools with double-ended brushes, tools whose bristles stiffly scratch, and tools whose tufts tenderly caress. There is a proper tool for every little nook and cranny of the body, and a proper way to use each one.

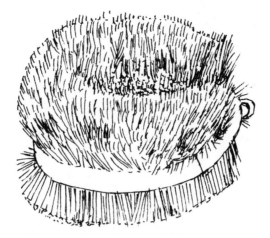

Starting with the softest and ending with the hardest, the following list describes some of the scrubbers and polishers available. Because those composed of natural materials are plentiful and appealing, the list does not include synthetic scrubbing tools, although these tools are often efficient and attractive as well.

The Sea Sponge, the Milk Sponge, the Devil's Tongue Root Sponge, the Silk Mitt or Bag

These are the softest and finest body-polishers, appropriate for the most sensitive, delicate complexions or for bathing young babies. Even when rubbed briskly over the skin, these will never irritate. Except for the tenderest and fairest of skins, these scrubbers are too soft for thorough body exfoliation and stimulation.

The *Tenugui* Towel, the Cotton Bag or Mitt

The *tenugui* is a small elongated rectangle of fine cotton, about the size of a Western face towel. The *tenugui* is used for a variety of purposes in Japanese life, and has traditionally been used in the bath, either as is or sewn into a bag to be filled with cleansing powder. The *tenugui* and the cotton bag or mitt are good basic face and body polishers; they are only slightly rough-textured, so they wash efficiently and exfoliate gently. These may be used by every skin type and on every part of the body.

The Facial or Complexion Brush

This small soft-textured brush is designed for the face. Handled or not, this type of brush is similar to a man's shaving brush, sometimes a bit stiffer. The bristles are always flexible. The facial brush may irritate sensitive skins, and for any skin type, proper technique is essential to avoid damage. Using very small circular motions, the brush is gently stroked over the face, always wet and with some kind of cleanser. The brush is an efficient stimulator and exfoliator, but care must be taken not to scrub overzealously. The facial brush is not useful for other body areas, as it is too small and too soft.

153

The Abrasive Towel, the Abrasive Sponge, the Loofah Sponge, the Hemp Friction Mitt or Strap, the Hemp Brush

These tools, all designed for body use, are rough-textured and somewhat stiff. The effect of these scrubbers will vary according to the pressure applied. These are generally too coarse for use on the face, though some soft loofahs or abrasive sponges or towels may be employed if handled with extreme delicacy. The abrasive towel is usually the same size and shape as the *tenugui,* but woven with coarser material, with a rougher texture. This type of towel is very useful for scrubbing one's own back, due to its length. The loofah, known in Japan as *hechima,* is a popular scrubber in many parts of the world. A natural gourd-fiber sponge, the loofah is somewhat absorbent and quite flexible when wet, thus it is convenient for use with cleansing ingredients or soap. The long-size loofah is good for back-scrubbing, but a bit unwieldy for general use.

The Hard-Backed Scrubbing Brush

There are many types of hard-backed brushes, and much variation in texture, size, and design. Those with detachable handles or which may be fitted with back-washing straps are most practical. Palm-size hard-backed brushes are designed for use on the body, never the face.

The *Tawashi* Scrubbing Brush

This stiff brush looks a lot like a vegetable scrubber, and in fact is originally a kitchen brush. The *tawashi* is all bristle, without a hard back, and comes in various sizes and degrees of firmness. The smallest is about the size of a lemon, the largest the size of a papaya. The hardest *tawashi* is made of palm-shell fibers, with hemp palm and hemp composing the softer versions. The *tawashi* is a good basic scrubber for most of the body, but it may be too abrasive for breasts, inner arms, and inner thighs. It should never be used on the face!

The Pumice Stone

The volcanic pumice stone—or lightweight-rock *karuishi,* as it's called in Japanese, is a familiar presence on Japanese beaches and in Japanese baths. The pumice stone is used on the toughest, roughest callused areas—feet, knees, and elbows. A faithful daily rub with the *karuishi* gives quick results: silky-smooth heels, feet that gleam like mother-of-pearl, and softly polished knees and elbows.

All brushes, bags, mitts, and sponges must be frequently cleansed with soap and hung to dry. If this is not done every few days, especially if the scrubbing tool remains damp in a warm environment, bacteria will proliferate rapidly.

Rice Bran Body Scrub

Actions:

Cleanses
Moisturizes
Softens
Smooths
Lightens
Heals

Indications:

All skin types
Daily use

Ingredients:

Fresh pure rice bran

Preparation:

Fill a body-scrubbing bag with finely ground rice bran, then soak the bag in warm water (in the bath is fine) until the bran is softened and a milky liquid begins to seep out.

Directions for Use:

Scrub and massage the body thoroughly with the rice bran bag, moistening it as needed in water.

Beautiful skin is as fine and white as the delicately gleaming grain of cooked white rice; as soft as a round white rice cake; as tender, as plump, as innocent, as generous, as fragrant . . . as rice. For rice-cake skin, it is to rice bran that the traditional woman turns, and the rice bran rewards her with polished skin of silky-smooth white, a skin of secret beauty, to be concealed beneath an equally silky kimono.

155

Bean and Bran Powder Scrub

Pink bean powder and rice bran, the two most beloved cleansing powders, are used in combination to polish the body to a satin glow. The powder of azuki beans has had a luxurious and aristocratic image since the eighth century, when women of noble birth used it to cleanse and beautify their skin; rice bran, being cheaper, more plentiful, and widely available, is a more democratic substance. One might say that putting these two together is a revolutionary act against the old class structure. The result is elegant and supremely functional.

Actions:

Cleanses
Exfoliates
Lightens
Softens
Moisturizes
Smooths
Heals
Stimulates

Indications:

All skin types
Daily use

Ingredients:

Azuki bean powder (see chapter on face washes for preparation method)
Rice bran

Preparation:

Mix equal amounts of rice bran and azuki bean powder, and place in a body-scrubbing bag.

Directions for Use:

Moisten the bag until a milky liquid emerges, then use it to scrub and massage the body thoroughly, remoistening the bag as needed.

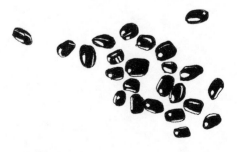

Stimulating Ginger-Root Scrub

Actions:

Cleanses
Purifies
Stimulates circulation
Warms
Eases aches and pains

Indications:

Not recommended for sensitive skin
Weekly use or as needed

Ingredients:

14 ounces (400 cc) fresh ginger root
8½ cups (2 liters) pure spring water

Preparation:

Grate the ginger. Add the ginger juice acquired from grating to the water in a nonmetal pot. Wrap the ginger solids in gauze and place this in the pot as well.

Boil the water for a minute or two, then allow to cool slightly. The water should be as hot as possible, but not so hot that one would be burned by touching it.

Directions for Use:

Dip a *tenugui* towel or small washing cloth into the hot ginger-water, then use it to scrub the body, dipping the towel repeatedly so that the liquid applied is always warm.

Hot and spicy ginger is used medicinally in a variety of ways. The combined action of the scrubbing massage with the stimulation of ginger makes this a deeply invigorating treatment. Not for daily use, but very good when one is fatigued or under the weather, the ginger-root scrub is a potent healing remedy for general malaise.

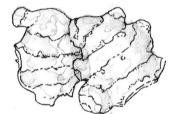

157

Seaweed Bath Scrub

In the aquamarine depths of
the undersea kingdom, it is
undoubtedly with soft green
seaweed that little sea princesses
wash their treasured selves. (To
complete the oceanic effect, ladle
generous quantities of sea salt
into your warm bath.)

Actions:

Cleanses
Stimulates
Detoxifies
Revives
Tones

Indications:

All skin types
Daily use or as frequently as desired

Ingredients:

Any dried edible sea plant without additives

Preparation:

Soften dried seaweed by soaking in tepid water
for 20 minutes.

Directions for Use:

Place seaweed in a washing bag—powdered
seaweed may be used in the same manner—
moisten in warm water, and use to scrub and
massage the body before and during bathing.

BODY TREATMENTS

A beautiful body requires beautiful skin. For this, the Japanese woman relies largely on good diet and the daily bath-soak-scrubbing ritual. For extra protection of the skin's moisture and prevention against dryness, roughness, or chapping, simple oils, emollients, or plant waters may be applied.

As an occasional all-over nourishing or revitalizing treatment, the same ingredients used on the face may be applied: black sugar, rice bran, egg whites, honey,

---

How to use body treatments:

Massages and Soaks
- may be carried out independent of bathing. Generally such treatments require no rinsing; this is a matter of personal preference.

Prebath Treatments
- may be applied just prior to bathing, or after washing and rinsing but before a bath-soak.

Postbath Treatments and Packs
- are applied after washing and soaking, when the skin is still moist and warm. The body must be kept warm during the treatment; in the case of a pack which is kept on for fifteen to thirty minutes, the reclining body may be covered with a heavy towel or a blanket. A sauna is a good place for such body treatments and packs. Most of the treatments in this category are rinsed.

Rinses and Pats
- are conveniently carried out at the end of the bathing process, as most are not meant to be rinsed.

Spot Treatments
- are mostly designed to be applied and reapplied repeatedly, without rinsing, though some are packs which are left on for a short period and then rinsed, and some are packs designed to be left on continuously.

bush warbler droppings, loofah vine water. To cool and soothe overheated, inflamed summer skin, or to warm, soften, and nourish the body chapped and chilled by winter, there are age-old remedies. There are simple plant remedies for purifying and healing rashes, blemishes, and irritated skin. The traditional remedies for banishing warts, corns, and calluses are sometimes—as in other cultures—touched with magic: for example, a big wart is invited to disappear by tying it at its base with a bit of silken thread.

Basic Camellia Nut Oil Body Care

Camellia nut oil, as the basic, all-around beauty oil, can be used in a variety of ways to nourish, soften, and protect the skin. For daily care of the body, apply a light coating of the oil all over before bathing. Another method is to apply the oil after bathing, followed by a little lemon juice—said to multiply the benefits of camellia oil—and then a final brisk toweling. The oil may also be added directly to the bathwater if preferred. These techniques will protect skin's moisture and keep it soft and smooth.

As a massage treatment for very dry areas, camellia nut oil may be mixed with honey or a commercial cream. Chapped hands and feet may be soaked in a basin of warm water with a few drops of oil. To lighten and soften the hands, massage warmed camellia nut oil into the skin and nails, wrap the hands in towels or put on cotton gloves for ten minutes, then remove the oil and apply lemon juice. Calluses and rough skin on the feet will be softened by applying the oil after rubbing with a pumice stone.

A good allover body treatment is the black sugar-camellia nut oil body pack. Apply the mixture everywhere after bathing and leave on for fifteen minutes. This will relieve sunburn and lighten and soften the skin.

Rice Bran Body Tonic

Actions:

Softens
Smooths
Nourishes
Moisturizes
Heals

Indications:

All skin types
Recommended for dry skin
Use daily

Ingredients:

4 cups (950 cc) rice bran
4 quarts (4 liters) water

Preparations:

Place rice bran in a cloth bag and add to water in a nonmetal pan. Bring to a boil and allow to boil for 15 minutes.

Leave the rice bran bag in the water to steep until it cools. Squeeze the bag into the water and remove it. (Save the bag to put in the bath.)

This rice bran water may be kept in the refrigerator for up to one week.

Directions for Use:

Rub the liquid over the freshly cleansed body after bathing. Rinsing is not necessary.

NOTE: This tonic can be used for basic daily care.

A light moisturizing tonic for the body can be made from the old Japanese favorite: rice bran.

Tofu Body Pack

Tofu has a healing, calming effect when used externally; it nourishes the skin with vitamins, minerals, protein, and light oil without being too rich or too stimulating.

Actions:

Aids healing
Lightens scars
Tones
Nourishes

Indications:

All skin types
Recommended for sensitive, irritated skin
Use occasionally

Ingredients:

2 blocks fresh tofu
Rice bran/rice flour

Preparations:

Squeeze tofu in a cloth to drain some of the liquid, then add a little rice bran or flour to stiffen it. The mixture should be made creamy by beating with a wooden spoon or mixing in a blender.

Directions for Use:

Apply the pack to freshly cleansed skin wherever toning and nourishment is needed. Leave the pack on for 15 minutes, then rinse off with cool water.

NOTE: Use as an occasional treatment or for special care.

Salty Pounded Turnip

Actions:

Purifies

Heals

Indications:

All skin types

Recommended for rashes and blemishes

Ingredients:

Raw turnip

Sea salt

Preparation:

Pulverize small chunks of turnip using a mortar and pestle. When the turnip is well mashed, add salt.

Directions for Use:

Apply the salty turnip mash to the area of inflammation for 15 to 20 minutes. Repeat as needed.

NOTE: Use as an occasional treatment or for special conditions.

For an all-out purification program, one may combine the salty turnip treatment with regular baths in sake, *the drinking of pearl barley or dokudami* tea, *and the eating of daikon radish,* umeboshi, *and garlic. Eating fruits rich in vitamin C is also beneficial.*

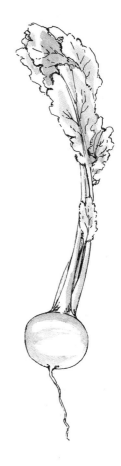

163

Loofah Vine Body Tonic

Hechimasui *is good for preserving and protecting the skin, without any of the inconveniences of an oil. The plant water acts to hold in moisture, and in the case of skin damage—chaps, cracks, burns, sunburns, heat rash—rapidly repairs and restores the skin to its natural silky beauty.*

164

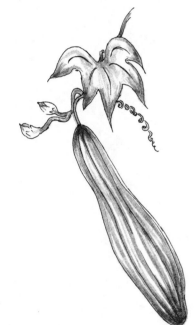

Actions:

Protects
Guards against moisture loss
Softens
Heals
Soothes

Indications:

All skin types
Recommended for the protection of skin exposed to cold, wind, or sun
Use daily

Ingredients and Preparation:

See the recipe for Loofah Vine Water in the section on facial waters.

Directions for Use:

Apply to the freshly cleansed body after bathing. Do not rinse.

NOTE: This tonic can be used for basic daily care.

Chilled Gauze-Wrapped Cucumber Tap

Actions:

Cools
Soothes
Softens
Smooths
Lightens

Indications:

Not recommended for sensitive or allergy-prone
  skin
Recommended for sunburn, overheated skin,
  blotches
Apply as needed

Ingredients:

One chilled cucumber

Preparation:

Grate the chilled cucumber and wrap in a square
of gauze.

Directions for Use:

Without squeezing the bag, tap it repeatedly and
gently over the skin.

Another method is to squeeze the bag to extract
juice, then pat the juice onto the skin.

No rinsing is required.

**NOTE: Use as an occasional treatment or for special
conditions.**

*This quick remedy offers an
elegant chill in the hot depths of
summer.*

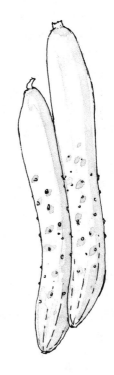

165

Ginger Water Massage

Winter—the time of dark days and cold nights. The old-fashioned wooden houses are so drafty that the Japanese have become adept in body-warming methods—the bath with tangerines or citrons, which warms the body and the spirit with fragrant bright yellow or orange fruits; warming stews and soups full of strengthening root vegetables such as diakon, carrots, and taro; and rich-flavored mushrooms, orange pumpkin, or balls of devil's tongue root. Winter is the time for hot sake and invigorating ginger kuzu tea, and for vitamin C, sweet tangerines from the southern islands or orange-red persimmons eaten fresh or chewy-dried. The nightly hot bath is a necessity—taken just before bedtime, the body soaks up the heat, ready to slide into a cozy futon with its thick soft quilts, while the snow falls silently outside.

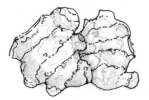

Actions:

Warms

Cleanses

Stimulates circulation

Eases muscle aches and joint pains

Invigorates

Indications:

Not recommended for children or those with sensitive skin

Recommended for winter chills or poor circulation

Use as needed

Ingredients:

Fresh ginger root

Hot water

Preparation:

Grate a big chunk of ginger, then squeeze through a cloth to obtain the juice, which is then added to a basin containing very hot water.

Directions for Use:

Dip a small towel into the ginger-water, wring well, and pat and rub the body with it. (This should be done in an extremely warm room—a bathing room full of warm steam is perfect.)

A clear-water rinse may be desired, especially if the skin is somewhat sensitive.

NOTE: Use as an occasional treatment or for special conditions.

Wasabi Massage

Actions:

Stimulates circulation
Warms
Destroys germs
Purifies

Indications:

Not recommended for children or those with
  sensitive skin
Recommended for winter chills or poor
  circulation
Use occasionally

Ingredients:

Fresh *wasabi* root, or *wasabi* powder or paste
Hot water

Preparation:

For the fresh root, grate with a very fine
ginger/*wasabi* grater.

Dilute the freshly ground *wasabi* or *wasabi*
powder or paste, with very warm water in a
basin (about a tablespoon of *wasabi* should be
adequate).

Directions for Use:

Massage the liquid into cold hands and feet.
Used over a period of time, this remedy is said
to improve circulation.

**NOTE: Use as an occasional treatment or for special
conditions.**

*As anyone who has ever eaten
sushi knows, wasabi is potent
stuff. This massage is worth
trying if all else fails to warm
you. It is wise to proceed with
extreme caution, and the highest
level of respect for this bitingly
hot green root.*

Honey-Lemon Treatment

A sweet-and-sour skin softener.

Actions:

Softens rough skin
Moisturizes
Lightens

Indications:

All skin types
Recommended for rough skin
Use occasionally

Ingredients:

Juice from 1 lemon
4 tablespoons (60 ml) honey

Preparation:

Mix the ingredients.

Directions for Use:

Apply to a freshly cleansed body and leave on for 15 minutes, then rinse with cool water.

NOTE: Use as an occasional treatment or for special conditions.

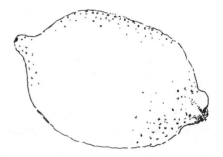

Seaweed Body Pack

Actions:

Stimulates cell functions
Tones
Heals
Purifies
Regenerates
Nourishes

Indications:

All skin types
Recommended for skin that needs toning
Use as needed

Ingredients:

Wakame seaweed (*Undaria pinnatifida*)

Preparation:

Fresh *wakame* should be soaked briefly in warm water, then rinsed to remove salt. Dried *wakame* must be soaked in warm water for 20 minutes for softening prior to use.

Directions for Use:

After thoroughly scrubbing and cleansing the body, apply the seaweed strips all over the body or on particular areas. It is best to cover the body completely and then recline for 30 minutes. After removal of the seaweed, rinse with cool water.

NOTE: Use as an occasional treatment or for special conditions.

This is the kind of regenerating, revitalizing, cell-activating treatment that people journey to exclusive spas for. One does need a place to stretch out seaweed-wrapped, and perhaps a helper to aid in the application of the long green strips, whose deep-sea nutrients will bring an extraordinary sparkle and tone to the skin.

169

Whipped Egg-White Body Pack

Someday when you've got huge numbers of extra egg whites, whip them up into a stiff mountain and—go ahead, it's fun—cover every inch of your bare body with them. Aside from transforming you into a fantasy snow-creature, the treatment will soften all your skin's rough spots.

Actions:

Softens
Tones
Tightens

Indications:

All skin types
Recommended for rough skin
Use occasionally

Ingredients:

Lots of egg whites

Preparation:

Whip egg whites until stiff.

Directions for Use:

Apply evenly to a freshly cleansed body, leave for 15 minutes, then rinse with cool water.

NOTE: Use as an occasional treatment or for special conditions.

VANISHING RECIPES
(FOR CALLUSES, WARTS, AND CORNS)

The calyx of the **eggplant** is the part of the stem which spreads out like an elf-hat where it is attached to the vegetable. For warts, this calyx is rubbed on them faithfully until they gradually vanish.

White **fig stem sap**, which seeps from a cut fig leaf, stem, or branch, is applied daily to warts, corns, and calluses. If the skin is irritated by this stem sap, first apply a paste of kneaded boiled white rice to the spot, then put the sap on top of the rice.

Black sugar syrup is made by boiling unrefined dark sugar with pure water. It may be applied to callused areas—feet, elbows, and knees—left on to work for a few minutes, and then rinsed off. Said to be exfoliating and softening, the black sugar will gradually smooth and refine coarse, hardened skin.

The white milk from the stem of the **dandelion** may be applied to warts several times daily until they disappear.

Pearl barley is a high-powered wart remedy that combines both internal and external treatments. Grind pearl barley seeds to a fine powder, then mix three teaspoons of the powder with water to form a creamy paste. Simmer the mixture for a few minutes, eat half of it, apply the rest to the wart (making a bandage to hold it in place), and continue the treatment for ten days. The same treatment is said to lighten age spots and freckles.

With the exception of black sugar syrup, the vanishing recipes may cause irritation to some skins. Sensitive skins and young skins should abstain; anyone using these remedies should discontinue use if redness, inflammation, or irritation develops.

The drinking of **pearl barley** tea and the eating of pearl barley cream porridge should accompany any wart-removal program.

VITALIZING TEAS AND TONICS

*T*he presence of energy, vitality, or *ki* is primary to the beauty, health, and harmony of the body. When one feels good in one's skin (or *bien dans sa peau*, as the French would say) one has the sense that the vital energy flow is smooth, harmonious; everything is in good working order and balance. The teas and tonics presented here are chosen for their properties of strengthening, vitalizing, and toning. When the diet is basically sound, these beverages can serve as energizing, health-promoting supplements.

Along with the benefits to overall body condition, some of the drinks described may be used to encourage the regulation of weight, to eliminate toxins, quickly relieve fatigue, and improve resistance to illness. Many of the drinks serve as both prevention and cure; they are gentle medicines that enable the body to maintain energy and health.

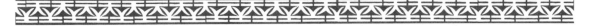

Roast Rice Bran Tea

Actions:

Nourishes
Revitalizes

Indications:

Recommended for improvement of general
   condition
Take daily

Ingredients:

1 tablespoon (15 cc) rice bran
½ cup (120 ml) pure spring water

Preparation:

Roast rice bran for 1 to 2 minutes over a
medium flame, stirring constantly.

Stir into the tepid water.

Directions for Use:

Drink.

*Rice bran works for beauty from
the inside too.*

173

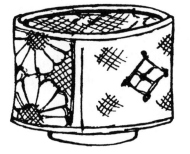

Roast Barley Tea

An everyday Japanese scene during the hot, hot summertime: mothers and children sit in the shade drinking ice-cold mugi-cha, barley tea. The tea has a delicious smoky-clear flavor, and is said to be cleansing and fat-eliminating, as well as refreshing.

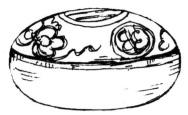

Actions:

Combats water retention
Eliminates toxins and fats
Cleanses
Refreshes

Indications:

Recommended for use on weight-loss programs or for relief from heat
Take daily

Ingredients:

4 tablespoons (60 cc) barley
2½ cups (600 ml) pure spring water

Preparation:

Roast barley in a heavy skillet for 5 minutes over a medium flame, stirring constantly.

Add barley to water in a nonmetal pan, bring to a boil, then lower to a simmer for 10 minutes. Filter to remove barley.

May be stored in the refrigerator for several days.

Directions for Use:

Drink the tea hot or cold. Avoid drinking copious amounts or giving it to children in large quantities—it is a diuretic tea.

Shiitake Mushroom Tea

Actions:

Relaxes
Stimulates diuresis
Reduces cholesterol

Indications:

Recommended for stress
Take once daily

Ingredients:

One shiitake mushroom, fresh or dried
2 cups (480 ml) pure spring water
Sea salt

Preparation:

If using a dried mushroom, soak in warm water for 30 minutes or until soft.

Slice the mushroom, add to the water with a pinch of salt in a nonmetal pan, then bring to a boil, lowering heat to a simmer for 15 minutes.

Directions for Use:

Sip slowly, taking only a small amount of the tea at a time.

Many of the Japanese so-called teas, like this mushroom one, should perhaps be thought of as broths. Somehow, placing the salty, seaweed, root, or fungus-based liquids in the soup category rather than the beverage group makes them seem more palatable—especially to the Westerner, for whom drinks are more likely to be sweet than salty or savory.

Garlic Tonic

Garlic is said to possess antibiotic properties, improve sexual stamina, beautify the skin, clean the blood, stimulate the metabolism, make the hair strong and shiny, regenerate cells, revive, encourage the elimination of wastes, toxins, and excess water, make swelling go down, get rid of skin problems, clear the arteries of cholesterol, relieve colds and coughs, rev up all body functions, and guard against disease. Need one say more?

176

Actions:

Improves all functions
Strengthens
Purifies
Vitalizes

Indications:

Recommended as a general tonic
Take daily

Ingredients:

2 cups (500 cc) fresh garlic
31 ounces (0.9 liter) *shochu* or vodka

Preparation:

Peel and slice the garlic, then place it in a clean glass bottle with alcohol, to be stored well sealed in a cool, dark location for one year.

Directions for Use:

Drink a tablespoonful of the tonic every day.

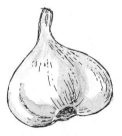

Ginseng Tonic

Actions:

Tones the system
Vitalizes
Relieves fatigue
Improves resistance

Indications:

Recommended as a general tonic
Take daily

Ingredients:

1 large dried ginseng root, or several small roots
31 ounces (0.9 liter) *shochu* or vodka

Preparation:

Wash root with a brush; dry. Tie ginseng root with a cord and suspend it from the neck of the bottle so that it is "standing up" in the bottle, with its roots just touching the bottom. Add alcohol, seal the lid with wax, then store in a dark cool location for one year.

Directions for Use:

Drink 1 *sake*-size cupful of the tonic nightly.

Soon after arriving in Japan I was excited to discover that the local corner store sold small bottles of ginseng drink, right next to canned tea and Coke in the refrigerator. When I bought a bottle of it, I couldn't understand why the shop-owner burst into uncontrollable giggles and turned bright red. Later, I learned that the drink is for men only, taken specifically to improve sexual endurance. My husband was getting embarrassed looks for months.

This tea is a highly nutritious beverage that tastes like hay, is an invigorating bright spring green, and is more immediately stimulating than a cup of French roast coffee.

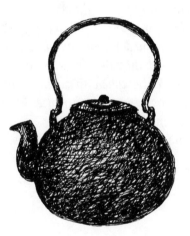

178

Actions:

Nourishes
Energizes
Tones the system

Indications:

Recommended for fatigue, stress, and poor condition
Take daily

Ingredients:

Powdered dried young barley grass (marketed as Green Magma in the West)
Pure spring water

Preparation:

Add a teaspoonful of the powder to a glass of tepid water and stir.

Directions for Use:

Drink.

Chinese Black Tea

Actions:

Cleanses
Eliminates fat
Eliminates excess water

Indications:

Recommended for use by those on slimming
   regimes
Take daily

Ingredients:

1 teaspoon (5 cc) oolong or *polei* tea
¾ cup (180 ml) pure spring water

Preparation:

Add just-boiled water to the tea in a teapot;
steep 1 to 2 minutes.

Directions for Use:

Drink.

The Chinese fermented teas—the black teas— oolong and polei *(or bolei) are the favorite teas among Japanese women on slimming regimes. These teas are said to dissolve and wash away fat, always a pleasant thought to anyone who feels too rounded. There is some controversy as to whether the teas actually melt fat, but these are the teas used by sumo wrestlers when they retire and want to slim down.*

179

Sweet Spirits of Aloe

Aloe gel makes a popular health drink in Japan—some use a juicer to combine aloe, lemon, parsley, and carrot juice for a daily health-maintenance drink. This recipe is more old-fashioned.

Actions:

Protects health
Improves resistance
Soothes

Indications:

Recommended to improve general condition
Take daily

Ingredients:

10 ounces (300 cc) fresh aloe leaves
½ cup (120 cc) black sugar or rock sugar
24 ounces (720 ml) *shochu* or vodka

Preparation:

Wash the leaves, dry well, then slice them into finger-length pieces. Place them in a clean glass jar with sugar and alcohol, seal tightly, then store in a cool, dark location for three weeks.

Remove the aloe, seal the jar once more, and return it to the same location for another three months before using.

Directions for Use:

Drink a small amount—about 1 tablespoonful—daily.

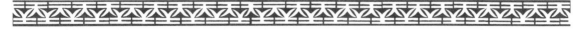

Sea Pearl Tea

Actions:

Calms
Eliminates toxins
Purifies

Indications:

Recommended for stress
Take as needed

Ingredients:

1 teaspoon (5 cc) powdered pearl
½ cup (120 ml) warm spring water or green tea

Preparation:

Stir powdered pearl into warm water or tea.

Directions for Use:

Sip slowly.

Asians have been drinking and eating pearls for centuries, not only for the calcium, but also for the pearl's pleasant ability to calm the nerves, relieve headaches, and induce sleep.

181

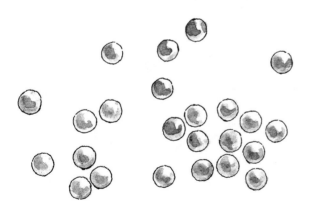

Ancient Algae Tea

Chlorella is 2 billion years old, but its use as a health drink is not so ancient. This microscopic green algae might be called the original detoxifier—it was one of the first green plants on Earth in the long ago days when the atmosphere was being transformed from a mixture of deadly gases into something more accommodating to higher forms of life. This algae is said to possess properties that help eliminate toxins, particularly hydrocarbons, heavy metals, and pesticides. Scientists are in the process of studying its potential use in preventing disease and signs of aging.

182

Actions:

Detoxifies
Nourishes

Indications:

Recommended for improving overall condition
Take daily

Ingredients:

Chlorella powder
Pure spring water

Preparation:

Stir a tablespoonful or so of chlorella powder into a glass of tepid water.

Directions for Use:

Drink.

Black Sugar Drink

Actions:

Relieves fatigue
Warms
Nourishes
Revives

Indications:

Recommended for fatigue
Take once daily or as needed

Ingredients:

1 tablespoon (15 cc) unrefined sugar (molasses
  may substitute)
1 cup (240 ml) hot spring water

Preparation:

Stir sugar or molasses into hot water.

Directions for Use:

Drink warm.

With the sugar for energy, and the rich array of vitamins and minerals for nourishment, this is a drink to take when one needs stimulation of a pleasantly sweet nature.

Pink Plum Bancha

This sounds like something sweet, but it is infinitely sour, like all umeboshi items. The umeboshi is the *everyday Japanese tonic food*, and this is *a pleasant way to take in its medicinal magic*.

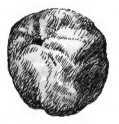

Actions:

Cleanses
Strengthens
Purifies
Revives
Relieves fatigue
Stimulates circulation
Cleans blood

Indications:

Recommended as a general tonic
Take daily

Ingredients:

1 teaspoon (5 cc) *bancha* tea
2 cups (480 ml) pure spring water
1 *umeboshi* (pickled plum)

Preparation:

Prepare *bancha* tea by boiling water and pouring it over the tea leaves in a teapot. Steep for 10 minutes.

Directions for Use:

Pour the tea into a cup, then add the crushed flesh of the *umeboshi*; drink.

Apricot Longevity Tonic

Actions:

Strengthens
Protects
Increases resistance
Vitalizes

Indications:

Recommended as a general tonic
Take daily

Ingredients:

4 cups (1 kilo) fresh apricots
3½ cups (800 cc) black sugar or rock sugar
7½ cups (1.8 liters) *shochu* or vodka

Preparation:

Wash, dry, and slice the apricots in two; do not discard/remove the pits. Place all ingredients in a clean glass bottle, seal tightly, and store in a cool, dark location. After two or three months, remove the fruits (one may eat them, boiled with some sugar).

Directions for Use:

Drink about 1 tablespoonful daily.

This medicinal tonic contains the potent benefits of the pit of the pretty apricot, which is reputed to keep one alive for a long, high-spirited lifetime.

THE BODY-CARE RITUAL

Daily

Morning: Cleanse the body in the shower; attend to hair and face routines.

After rinsing and drying, but while the body is still slightly damp, apply basic oil, emollient, or plant water.

Evening: Prepare the bath by filling the tub and adding whatever bath ingredient is desired.

Wash, scrub, and rinse thoroughly.

Soak in the bath for twenty minutes or so (with or without intermittent scrubbing sessions).

After rinsing and drying, apply basic oil, emollient, or plant water.

Weekly or As Needed

Morning or Evening: If using a prebath treatment, apply to the body while the tub is filling.

Wash, scrub, and rinse thoroughly.

Soak in the bath with or without intermittent scrubbing sessions.

Apply a body pack or special treatment and recline in a warm place, covered if necessary.

Return to the shower and rinse.

After rinsing and drying, apply basic oil, emollient, or plant water.

The face-care and hair-care routines are designed to be interwoven with the body-care routine as seems practical. Teas and tonics may be incorporated according to personal preference. Daily exercise activity, which includes attention to breathing, flexibility, strength, and endurance, is another important aspect of the total body-beauty ritual.

BODY REGIMENS

A personal body-care regimen may be designed by choosing à la carte from among the recipes in each section. Select a bath, a scrub and/or a scrubbing tool or tools, a daily oil, emollient, or plant water, a special treatment or body pack, and a tea or a tonic drink. Recipes may be chosen to benefit either skin-surface body conditions or total-body conditions (fatigue, poor circulation, postexercise muscle aches, etc.). The following regimens suggest appropriate programs for some common short-term and long-term, skin-surface and total-body conditions and needs.

Basic Maintenance for Any Skin
Rice Bran Bath
Brush Scrub/Rice Bran Body Scrub
Camellia Nut Oil
Seaweed Body Pack
Roast Rice Bran Tea

Dry Skin
Rice Bran Bath
Loofah Scrub/Rice Bran Body Scrub
Camellia Nut Oil
Honey Lemon Treatment
Roast Rice Bran Tea

Sensitive or Young Skin
Bath of Spring Rose Petals
Silk Mitt/Sea Sponge Scrub/Powdered Pearl Wash
Rice Bran Body Tonic
Tofu Body Pack
Black Sugar Drink

Aging Skin
Tonic Seaweed Bath
Brush Scrub/Seaweed Bath Scrub
Camellia Nut Oil
Seaweed Body Pack
Apricot Longevity Tonic

Irritated Skin
Yellow Chrysanthemum Bath
Sea Sponge Scrub/Rice Bran Body Scrub
Rice Bran Body Tonic
Tofu Body Pack
Roast Barley Tea

Sunburned Skin
Alkaline Bath
Seaweed Bath Scrub/No Scrub
Rice Bran Body Tonic
Chilled Gauze-Wrapped Cucumber Tap
Young Barley Grass Tea

To Calm Stressed Skin
December Citron Bath
Silk Mitt Scrub/Powdered Pearl Wash
Rice Bran Body Tonic
Tofu Body Pack
Shiitake Mushroom Tea

To Revitalize Tired Skin
Bath of Ginseng Root
Brush Scrub/Stimulating Ginger Root Scrub
Camellia Nut Oil
Seaweed Body Pack
Garlic Tonic

To Prevent or Treat Cellulite or to Accompany a Weight-Regulation Program
Tonic Seaweed Bath
Brush Scrub/Seaweed Body Scrub
Camellia Nut Oil
Seaweed Body Pack
Chinese Black Tea

To Relieve Tension, Stress, or Fatigue
Skin-Like-a-Gleaming-Jewel Rice Wine Bath
Brush Scrub/Rice Bran Body Scrub
Camellia Nut Oil
Ginger Water Massage
Apricot Longevity Tonic

To Invigorate, Revive, and Stimulate Circulation
Ginger Bath
Brush Scrub/Seaweed Bath Scrub
Camellia Nut Oil
Seaweed Body Pack
Garlic Tonic

To Cool and Refresh
Bath of Rice Vinegar
Seaweed Bath Scrub
Seaweed Body Pack
Iced Roast Barley Tea

To Warm
Ginger Bath
Brush Scrub/Stimulating Ginger Root Scrub
Ginger Water Massage
Black Sugar Drink

THE SUBLIME DETAIL

Anyone who participates in the Japanese tea ceremony, walks through a Japanese garden, or sits down to even the simplest of Japanese meals will notice the attention to detail. It is the smallest detail, focused on with complete concentration, a sense of care and precision, and the respect for the detail's innate subtlety, that offers stunning purity and charm to much that is Japanese. The unique Japanese harmony is created through the preservation of a gentle balance between the defined and refined details in the overall arrangement.

The same principle is at work in woman's beauty. In making herself up, the woman applies translucent, quiet color tones to her face, delineating and drawing to soft perfection the eyes, eyebrows, cheeks, lips, and complexion. No detail is neglected, yet the face remains understated, harmonious, and natural-looking. Individual features and colors do not vie with one another for attention. The makeup itself is barely discernible, though its unmistakable polish is present.

The same detailed focus applies to grooming. Along with the obvious complexion-cleansing and care, even the smallest aspects of the appearance receive diligent and loving attention. Downy hairs on the neck and face are shaved; the hairline is neatened, trimmed, and smoothed. The ears, softened with oil, are religiously scraped clean of wax and dusted. Teeth are brushed after every meal in a carefully orchestrated ritual of comprehensive cleansing and polishing. When eyes are tired, a few minutes are taken to cool them, bathe them, or simply close them for a momentary nap. Eyebrows are combed, polished, and shaped. The final impression is one of highly perfected naturalness.

ELEGANT EXTREMITIES

The hands and the feet, though less immediately obvious than face or hair, are nonetheless essential elements in the overall impression of elegant feminine beauty. Although one may not have been born with small, delicate, fair-complexioned hands and feet, with attentive grooming and graceful gestures it is possible to produce a truly lovely, refined effect.

The Japanese girl learns to hold her hands with quiet restraint, with a smallness and gentleness of movement that causes them to appear tinier and softer then they may indeed be. At rest, hands are held unobtrusively, fingers close together and curled slightly inward, resting one hand atop the other like nesting seashells or sleeping birds. In movement, too, there is control, an economy of gesture, a hint of shyness and delicacy, with a subtle bend of the exposed wrist, a slight rounding of the hand and fingers, with fingertips together, tapering. Such detailed attention to the hands may appear almost theatrical when compared with the average Western woman's hand movements, but it is merely the difference between a hand that is trained—like a dancer's—and one that is not.

The feet, too, are handled with restraint, with a rather stylized smallness and daintiness of movement that is the result of years of childhood training. In earlier times, the wearing of the kimono instructed the body directly in the feminine art of movement: walking, sitting, and standing were necessarily executed with the utmost grace, the legs enclosed as they were in the narrow kimono. Even now, though liberated from the kimono's restraints, girls are trained from their earliest years to sit with legs parallel, feet together, and to walk quietly. One rarely sees the vigorous wide strides common to modern Western women.

The beautiful hand is soft-skinned and white, with unobtrusive nails that are cut to medium-length, neither long nor short, and oval in shape. The beautiful feminine foot shares the same attributes. Traditional Japanese preference tends toward hands that are delicate and weak-looking rather than sturdy, and toward narrow, slender-toed feet.

Since ancient times, Japanese women have given careful attention to their fingernails, which were kept neatly trimmed, buffed, and shaped, then tinted a subtle translucent red with natural vegetable dye: the red of the safflower, also used for lips and cheeks; the juice of the red blossom of the garden balsam; or the scarlet sap from the stalk of the *dokudami*. The very natural quiet glow of red was in harmony with the understated Japanese aesthetic. Western-type nail polish, which arrived in Japan during the Meiji era, seemed vulgar by comparison: too shiny, too obvious, too artificial. The traditional nails were a suggestion, while the new Western nails were a statement. Even in present-day Japan, women with brightly polished nails are considered to be lacking in refinement and good breeding. Many women do not apply polish at all, or if they do, it is in a shade that is natural, matte, or translucent.

One Japanese practice that has begun to be popular in other parts of the world is nail-sloughing. With a very fine-toothed padded emery board, the surface of the nail is sloughed, removing stains, ridges, and old hard nail, followed by a seconded buffing to refine the polished surface. The final step consists of a high-polishing rub with a chamois buff-board and a polishing cream. The result of the treatment is nails that are a natural delicate rose tint, as shiny as pale pink seashells, and satin-smooth. These naturally pink-polished nails will require a touch-up only when significant portions of new nail appear, at which time the

Steps in the care of hands and feet

- Remove calluses and hard, rough skin during the scrubbing session that precedes a soak in the bath. Rubbing a natural pumice stone in small circles repeatedly over such areas will eventually give good results if practiced daily.
- A small nail brush is not only a good way to clean fingernails and toenails, but is also stimulating to these areas.
- Apply treatments, oils, or emollients *after* a soak in the bath. Or, one can do this during a bath, by applying whatever treatment is preferred, and letting hands and feet emerge from the bath while one soaks.
- After rinsing a treatment pack from hands and feet, apply oil or emollient while massaging, concentrating on areas of rough skin, calluses, and the nails and cuticles. Push the cuticles back with a cotton swab.
- Trim, clip, or file nails to the desired shape.

Camellia Oil and Rice Bran (Daily Care)

A gentle daily scrub of hands and feet with the rice bran bag (which will cleanse, lighten, nourish, and protect the skin) followed by a few drops of camellia oil applied directly to the nails and cuticles after bathing, then rubbing one's lightly oiled hands over hands and feet, will suffice as the basic daily ritual. Cuticles may be pushed back with a cotton swab after applying oil.

Black Sugar, Lemon, and Camellia Oil Treatments (Weekly Care)

To soften rough skin, lighten the complexion, and moisturize, use a weekly application of camellia oil mixed with either black sugar syrup or the fresh lemon juice. Whichever mixture is chosen, it should be massaged well into the hands and feet, then left on for twenty minutes to work. Best applied during or after a bath, the treatment mixture must be rinsed with clear warm water, but not washed with soap.

process is repeated, but only to the new nail growth. (To repeat the sloughing in the same area can lead to dangerously thin nails.) Both fingernails and toenails may be sloughed and polished in this manner.

Nails are beautiful only in a beautiful setting, and basic hand and foot care is simple enough. Essential steps are to remove callused skin, to soften rough or dry skin, to lighten skin if desired, to moisturize, and to protect. A pumice stone, some camellia oil, a little black sugar syrup, a fresh lemon, and perhaps a bag of rice bran will suffice nicely.

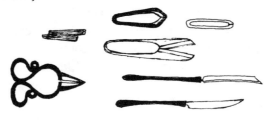

SCENT

There is an ancient Japanese tradition in the use of incense—both burning and nonburning varieties—as an aromatic, used to perfume clothing and hair, and to waft subtly upon the atmosphere of the home. Based on such fragrant woods as sweet pine, cinnamon, sandalwood, camphor, and Japanese yew, aromatic plants and spices such as clove, fennel, and licorice root, and such animal and mineral scents as musk and the powder of the spiral shell, Japanese fragrances are subtle and interesting, rarely sweet or heavy, never overbearing.

Western-style perfumes appeared in Japan during the Meiji era, attracting attention and achieving some measure of chic, but were never wholeheartedly embraced by Japanese women. Over the centuries the Japanese had developed a highly refined sense of fragrance; what is referred to in Japanese as "listening to a scent" was considered an important faculty for cultivated individuals to possess. The brighter, more aggressive nature of foreign perfumes and colognes must have been overwhelmingly loud. Lacking in them was the quiet, mysterious subtlety which is central to the Japanese sense of beauty, and which lends itself particularly well to the realm of fragrance—fragrance being at its most evocative when it exists as nothing more than an emanation, a suggestion, almost a feeling.

Incense occupies a domain encompassing magic, religion, ancestor spirits, gods, seduction, sex, poetry, memory, fashion, ritual purification, celebration, prayer, and the meditative state. The ability of incense/scent to penetrate and disperse, to exist palpably but invisibly, gives it a kind of transdimensional quality; in Japan as in many parts of the world, incense is thought to open a direct channel between the human realm and the unseen realms, where reside variously, gods, ancestor spirits, and the good, protective guardian spirits that stave off evil.

A recurring image in early Japanese literature is the one of incense burning while one awaits a lover; the passing of time marked by the burning down of the incense eases the difficulty of waiting. The fragrant smoke creates an atmosphere of charm and spirit, and also gives direct evidence of the passing of time. There were once fragrance clocks, containers for burning incense with smoke-openings marked for time periods, so that when smoke drifted through a particular opening the time could be thus read.

To perfume one's kimono was once de rigeur, and to this end there were several methods. One way was to burn incense placed within a *fusego,* a specially designed reversed basket attached to the top of an incense burner. Above this a kimono-smoking rack was erected, upon which the kimono was placed. This quick method for perfuming clothing was considered less refined than the smokeless *kakekou* method. The *kakekou,* a silk brocade drawstring sachet within which may be fragrant woods and barks, chopped aromatic grasses or crushed leaves, a kneaded paste composed of such substances, or a blend of fragrant powdered herbs, would be placed in a closet or clothing trunk, to lightly permeate stored apparel with scent.

A delightful effect was achieved by wearing scent bags, tucked into either bodice or obi, or two bags attached to either end of a cord worn draped around the neck, each bag concealed within a kimono sleeve.

As anyone knows who has spent even a few minutes in a smoky room, the hair seems to have an affinity for smoke, absorbing its aroma readily. Taking advantage of this natural propensity, Japanese women of earlier times perfumed their hair with the smoke from burning incense. Hair thus scented possesses a soft but rich fragrance that no liquid perfume can duplicate.

In old Japan, women would scent their tresses while they slept, with the head resting upon a high porcelain or lacquered wood pillow, with openings in its top through which smoke from the incense burning within could escape. Not a comfortable technique for the modern woman to adopt, the same effect may be achieved by allowing the smoke from an exquisite incense to drift into one's just-washed and still moist hair. The effect is sublimely sensual, with a natural, warm softness.

As described earlier in the book, essential oils and fragrances were used as ingredients in oils, emollients, pomades and cerates for both skin and hair. These were formulated so as to provide a whispered note of fragrance, vague and impalpable, like the feminine presence itself. To explore a Japanese feeling in scented oils, a few drops of essential oil may be added to an unscented carrier oil like camellia nut oil or safflower oil. Twenty-five drops of essential oil per 50 ml of carrier oil will supply a fragrant oil that may be used for face, hair, body, or bath. Pine, licorice root, clove, sandalwood, fennel, cinnamon, camphor, or borneol will lend a Japanese note.

The bath, of course, is another venue for imparting a light fragrance to the body. The bath of sweet flag; the citron or tangerine bath; the rose, chrysanthemum, perilla, honeysuckle, and ginger baths all leave a delicate waft of scent lingering about the bather.

When the first Western-style perfume arrived in Japan, publications advised women to make use of it by adding a few drops to a basin of water for washing the face and hands—noting, however, that Western women were apt to apply it not only directly to the skin but also to saturate their handkerchiefs with perfume, apply scented oils to their heads, and spray perfume directly onto their clothing. The general assumption was—and this idea persists to some extent—that all this perfuming was an attempt to cover up an unpleasant body odor, an affliction Westerners were thought to suffer.

Though the traditional forms of scent are widely available in Japan, as are Western perfumes, the Japanese woman who emanates an obvious fragrance is rare—indeed, she is likely to attract disapproving attention from among her peers for being too showy, lacking in taste and refinement. The Japanese claim to prefer the natural personal odor of a healthy, scrupulously clean, well-bathed body. When scent is applied, it is present in such minute amounts as to be practically imperceptible, at least to the untrained nose.

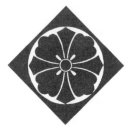

Daikon Deodorant

The giant white daikon radish is one of the most commonly used vegetables in Japanese cuisine. The daikon is employed both for its clean flavor and pleasant texture, whether cooked or raw, and for its purifying abilities. The daikon is said to purify when used externally too, which accounts for its use as an eliminator of odors.

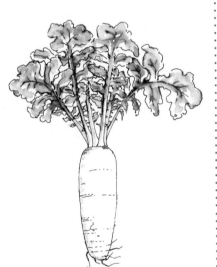

Actions:

Purifies

Eliminates odors

Indications:

Recommended as an underarm deodorant, for all skin types

Use daily

Ingredients:

Daikon radish

Preparation:

Using a daikon grater, grate a small piece of daikon, then squeeze the grated daikon through gauze to obtain the juice. Discard solids.

The juice may be kept refrigerated for 2 to 3 days.

Directions for Use:

After bathing, apply daikon juice to a cotton pad or cloth, then rub thoroughly into the underarm area.

Apply during the day as a refresher, as needed.

How to use incense:

1. To arrange incense items on a tray, the *kouro* (burner) must be placed at the top, the *koubako* (incense box) on the left, and the *koubashi* (incense chopsticks) on the right. Arrange them in a beautiful triangular shape.

2. The fire for the *kouro* must be made from *tadon* (charcoal briquettes). The *tadon* should be composed of a mixture of well-roasted walnut shells and pinecones, hardened with thin glue.

3. Form the ash into a lozenge shape. The proper number of times to press the ash is always an even number; an odd number is inauspicious.

4. When making *takimono* (room fragrance), one needn't press the ash. Instead *ginbon* (a mica tray trimmed with gold or silver leaf, placed between fire and incense for burning) may be used.

5. To make good *kakekou* (scent bags), one must learn how to mix aromatic substances in the right way. As an example, borneol, musk, clove, sweet pine, and sandalwood may be mixed together in proportions of 5:6:2:2:1.

   Kakekou containing *kyara* (Japanese yew) is especially nice. One can place *kakekou* between folded layers of kimono or hang it from a kimono hanger. In the hot summer season, one must take care that the *kakekou* fragrance is light. A too heavy scent lacks elegance. For kimono, *kyara* is the best scent to use. It would be best to permeate one's kimono directly while wearing it than to use a *fusego* (a basket reversed over an incense-burner) over which the kimono is draped.

From *Onna Chouhouki*, 1692
Translation by Michiko Kohama

197

Ten benefits of incense-burning:

Incense can move even a merciless god.

Incense can cleanse and purify one.

Incense removes poisons from one's body.

Incense can help one stay awake.

Incense can be a good friend when one is alone.

Incense can help one find moments of leisure even on the busiest days.

Incense may be used in large quantities.

Incense may be used in small quantities.

Incense may be kept for a long time, as it never goes bad.

Incense may be used every day.

Stated by Ikkyu, a priest of the Rinzai
sect of Buddhism in the Muromachi Era
Translation by Michiko Kohama

GRACE

The body becomes truly beautiful only through grace of expression: the way of speaking, the voice's tone and timbre, the facial expression, the look in the eyes all contribute. Grace is enduring where surface beauty is not. Grace is the direct expression of the inner nature, and as such may transcend the surface, making the most objectively nondescript face or body beautiful by supplying an atmosphere of harmony.

Grace might be best understood as consciousness: the mind present in the body, conscious of its effect upon others, conscious of its relationship to space. The controlled movements required by the wearing of certain garments are a form of externally induced body-consciousness. We are informed and created by the clothing we wear, by the spaces through which we move.

To cultivate grace is a simple matter: it occurs naturally, rising from within the moment we don an evening dress of fine silk, a kimono, or gauzy flowing skirts—any garment of great beauty to whose level we must rise with fluidity, softness, and femininity of movement.

APPENDIXES

JAPANESE HISTORICAL PERIODS

150,000 BC	Pre-Ceramic Culture
7000–300 BC	Jomon
300 BC–AD 300	Yayoi
300–710	Yamato
710–784	Nara
794–1185	Heian
1185–1333	Kamakura
1334–1395	Nambokucho
1392–1573	Muromachi
1573–1598	Azuchi-Momoyama
1603–1867	Edo
1868–1912	Meiji
1912–1925	Taisho
1926–1989	Showa
1989–	Heisei

A Guide to Preparations

HOW TO MAKE THE WASHING BAG

The accompanying illustration gives the basic pattern for the face-washing bag (small size) and the bath/body-scrubbing bag (large size). For both, 100 percent natural unbleached white silk or cotton should be used. In Japan a cotton *tenugui* towel is often used to make the large-size bath bag. (A long scrubbing bag, useful for back-washing, may be fashioned by sewing two *tenugui* towels together.)

To make either bag, two pieces of fabric cut to the dimensions indicated are sewn together on three sides, leaving an opening through which the scrubbing ingredients may be inserted. After filling, the bag is tightly tied shut with a cord, ready for use. Between uses, bags should be hung up to dry. Every few days, bags should be thoroughly laundered to keep them sanitary.

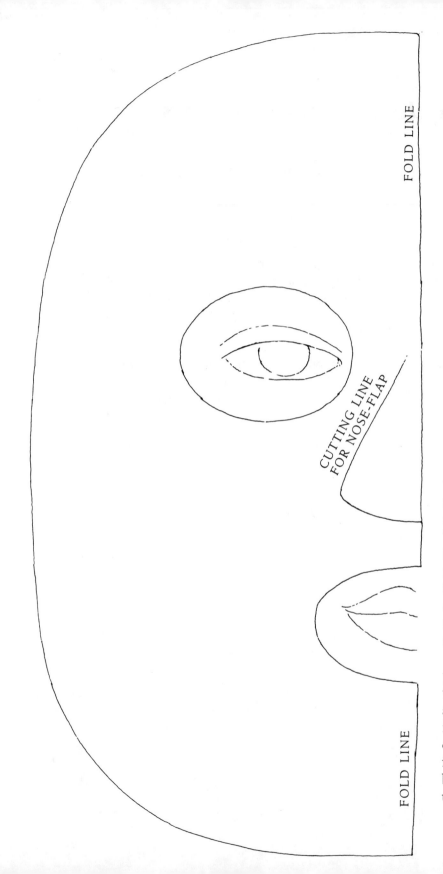

FOLD LINE

CUTTING LINE
FOR NOSE-FLAP

FOLD LINE

HOW TO MAKE THE FACE-PACK MASK

Use either very delicate rice paper—colorless and unbleached—or muslin, gauze, or cheesecloth. Make a pattern by tracing the half-mask illustrated and transferring the outline to a piece of cardboard. Fold the mask material and place the cardboard pattern over the folded rice paper or fabric, so that the center-face fold lines match. Draw the outline onto the material, then cut out. If the paper or fabric is thin enough, one can easily produce several masks simultaneously. It is a good idea to make enough face-pack masks to last for some time.

To use the mask, pour the pack liquid into a very shallow soup-bowl, as big or bigger than the mask. Then simply place the mask in flat and allow the liquid to penetrate it, then transfer it to the face, patting it smooth with a cloth. To remove, just peel the mask off from the forehead down.

For some nonliquid packs, particularly those which are thick but do not adhere well to the face, the face-pack mask is applied on top of the pack to help it remain in place. (It is best to lie down while using such packs.)

A Guide to Ingredients

MAIL-ORDER SOURCES FOR INGREDIENTS AND SUPPLIES

Aphrodisia
28 Carmine Street
New York, NY 10014
  Herbs of every description.

Atlantis Rising
7915 S.E. Stark
Portland, OR 97215
  Oriental herbs, oils, seeds.

Caswell-Massey Company
Catalog Order Department
320 West 13th Street
New York, NY 10014
  Basic ingredients for cosmetic-making, natural-bristle brushes and sponges.

Daniel Smith, Inc.
4130 1st Avenue South
Seattle, WA 91834
  Fine art supplies, including Japanese brushes and rice paper.

Diamond K Enterprises
R.R. 1, Box 30-A
St. Charles, MN 55972
TEL: 507-932-4308
  Organic foods.

Diamond Organics
Rockport, ME 04856
Freedom, CA 95019
TEL: 800-922-2396
  Organic produce, including tangerines, Chinese cabbage, wheat grass, *kabocha*, burdock root, daikon.

Frontier Direct
P.O. Box 127
Norway, IA 52318-0127
TEL: 800-726-5404
  Japanese and Chinese herbs and ingredients, essential oils, and supplies. Dried lotus pod, mugwort, apricot kernel oil, chrysanthemum blossoms, cassia, benzoin, sea plants, green and black teas, licorice root, plantain, safflower petals,

sandalwood, cherry bark, shiitake, dried burdock, chickweed, ginseng, mortars and pestles, small cotton bags, wide-necked jars, spice mills.

Garden Spot Distributors
Route 1, Box 729-A
New Holland, PA 17557
  Natural foods, including Japanese items.

George Ohsawa Macrobiotic Foundation
1511 Robinson Street
Oroville, CA 95965
TEL: 916-533-7702
  Japanese ingredients, books, supplies.

Gold Mine Natural Food Company
1947 30th Street
San Diego, CA 92102
TEL: 800-475-FOOD
  Macrobiotic and organic foods. Full line of top-notch Ohsawa America natural Japanese foods and ingredients. Eggplant toothpaste, burdock and *ume* concentrates, barley grass supplements, lotus root tea, green and black teas, *kuzu*, seaweeds, sea salt, black soybeans, azuki beans, all soybean products, dried daikon, mugwort, tofu, burdock, shiitake, brown rice vinegar, wasabi powder, pearl barley, rice bran, and more. Also offers Japanese Kitchen supplies.

The Green Earth
2545 Prairie
Evanston, IL 60201
TEL: 800-322-3662
  Organic produce, delivered anywhere in the U.S. Carries Chinese cabbage, burdock root, daikon, ginger, lotus root, *kabocha*, taro root.

Herb Products Company
11012 Magnolia Boulevard
North Hollywood, CA 81601
  Herbs, tinctures, essential oils, ginseng.

Maine Coast Sea Vegetables
Franklin, ME 04634
TEL: 207-565-2907
  Alaria, kelp, dulse, laver, seaweed
  seasonings, sea chips, seaweed candy. The
  company harvests and processes sea
  plants.

Mendocino Sea Vegetable Company
P.O. Box 372
Navarro, CA 95463
TEL: 707-895-3741
  Nori, alaria, *kombu*, dulse, flaked *nori*, and
  seaweed "feather boas" for the bath. The
  company harvests and processes sea
  plants.

Mountain Ark Trading Company
120 South East Avenue
Fayetteville, AR 72701
TEL: 800-643-8909
  Organic and macrobiotic Japanese foods,
  ingredients, and supplies. Mitoku foods,
  eggplant toothpaste, burdock concentrate,
  soybean products, sea plants, dried
  shiitake, bonito fish flakes, *ume* products,
  kuzu, pearl barley, green and black teas,
  sea salt, *wasabi* powder, *tawashi* scrub-
  brushes, 100% cotton cheesecloth, grain,
  seed, and coffee mills, graters, bamboo
  and wooden utensils, Japanese mortars
  and pestles and cutlery.

Natural Lifestyle Supplies
16 Lookout Drive
Asheville, NC 28804
  Macrobiotic ingredients and supplies.

Ohsawa America
440 Valley Drive
Brisbance, CA 94005
TEL: 800-475-3663
  Traditional, organic Japanese foods and
  macrobiotic items.

Organic Foods Express
11003 Emack Road
Beltsville, MD 20705
TEL: 301-937-8608
  Fresh organic produce, including daikon.
  Also oils, grains, seeds and nuts, flours,
  and other natural foods.

Paul's Grains
Rt. 1, Box 76
Laurel, IA 50141
TEL: 515-476-3373
  Organic grains, flours, and bran.

Shojin Natural Foods
Bhagavan Buritz
P.O. Box 669
Captain Cook, HI 96704

Starflower
885 McKinley Street
Eugene, OR 97402
  Organic foods and herbs.

Star Herb Company
38 Miller Avenue
Mill Valley, CA 94941
  Herbs and essential oils.

Walnut Acres
Penns Creek, PA 17862
TEL: 800-433-3998
  Organic and natural foods: whole grains,
  flours, high-quality oils, garlic capsules,
  kelp granules, molasses, honey, rice bran,
  and coffee, grain, and spice mills.

Whole Earth Access Company
Mail Order Department
2950 Seventh Street
Berkeley, CA 94710
  Food-preparation supplies and utensils.

Wide World of Herbs Ltd.
11 Saint Catherine Street East
Montreal 129
Quebec, Canada
  Unusual herbs and essential oils.

SAFETY PRECAUTIONS

Before making use of any ingredient with which one is not familiar, it is advisable to conduct a patch test to check for possible sensitivity. Make a paste by mixing the substance in question with a small amount of water, then apply a bit of this paste to the forearm, near the inner elbow crook. Hold the paste in position with a bandaid, to be kept in place for twenty-four hours. If after this time any redness, irritation, or inflammation is noticeable, it would be wise not to use the ingredient responsible. Among the substances known to occasionally produce allergic reactions or irritation in susceptible persons are the following:

Bergamot	Castor Oil	Lotus	Plantain
Buckwheat	Cucumber	Mugwort	Saffron
Camphor	Ginkgo	Mulberry	Strawberry
Cassia	Lemon	Orange	Tangerine

Taken internally, any of the kernels or kernel oils of peach, plum, or apricot are toxic in large doses.

LIST OF INGREDIENTS

For each ingredient mentioned in this book, its common English, Japanese, and Latin names are provided. If the item is used in the Chinese herbal medicine tradition, a Chinese name is often supplied as well. When the Chinese name is included, the order is as follows: English, Japanese, Chinese, Latin. The Latin botanical name may be useful in buying from either a Chinese or a Western herbalist.

For most ingredients, the part of the plant or substance that is employed in treatments is specified. For certain ingredients, especially those likely to be unfamiliar to Westerners, information on distinguishing characteristics, preparation, and storage requirements is supplied.

This guide lists single ingredients ordered alphabetically, with six listings containing grouped categories of closely related items: Fish and Seafoods; Plum ("Ume") Products; Rice and Rice Products; Sea Plants; Soybeans and Soybean Products; Tea. Ingredients mentioned only in passing and not included in any recipe have not been included in the guide.

Note: A fresh ingredient is equivalent to double or triple the volume of its dried form.

Aloe : Rokai : Lu Hui : Aloe Vera, A. Arborescens, A. Barbadensis (Liliaceae). Leaf gel. Fresh leaves may be wrapped in plastic and refrigerated. Available as a live plant at garden nurseries, as an extract at natural foods stores, herb stores, and Chinese medicine stores.

Apricot : Anzu : Xing Ren : Prunus Armeniaca L. (Rosaceae). Fruits and fruit kernels (fruit kernels are toxic in high doses). Available at all greengrocers as fruit in season; available in kernel or oil form at herb stores and Chinese medicine stores.

Azuki Beans : Azuki : Hong Tou : Phaseolus Species. Seeds. Azuki beans are small, shiny, dark red beans. Available at supermarkets and Japanese/Oriental markets.

Baking Soda : Juso or Itansan Suiso Natoryomu : Sodium Bicarbonate. Powdered mineral. Widely available.

Barley : O-Mugi : Mai Ya : Hordeum Vulgare (Graminae). Grains, dried germinated sprouts, which are *o-mugi wakaba* in Japanese. Available as a grain at supermarkets and natural foods stores and in barley grass or sprout form at natural foods stores.

Benzoin : Benzoin : Styrax Benzoin, S. Tonkinensis. Gum, tincture. Available at drugstores and herb stores.

Bergamot : Kankitsurui No Isshu : Citrus Bergamia. Fruit rinds and fruit rind oil. Available at herb stores as an oil.

Black Beans/Black Soybeans : Kuromame : Dou Chi : Glycine Max (Leguminosae). Seeds. These beans are black, somewhat larger than ordinary soybeans and shaped more like kidney beans. They are not identical to American black beans. Available at Japanese/Oriental markets and Chinese medicine stores.

Black Sugar : Kurozato : Saccharum officinarum. Sugar cane stem extract. This sugar is the least refined form of sugar, very dark brown, moist and chunky. It has a strong molasses-like aroma and taste, and molasses may substitute for it. Available at natural foods stores, Latin American markets, and Japanese/Oriental markets.

Buckwheat : Soba : Fagopyrum Esculentum. Seeds. Buckwheat causes allergic reactions in some people, used internally or externally. Available as seeds, groats, or flour at supermarkets, Japanese/Oriental markets, and natural foods stores.

Burdock/Great Burdock : Gobou : Ni Bang Zi : Arctium Lappa (Compositae). Roots, leaves, seeds. Burdock root is commonly around 2 feet/60 cm in length, tapering to a point from at its widest end, a diameter of 3/4 inches/2 cm.

Its rough brown skin should not be pared, but scrubbed with a stiff vegetable brush before preparation. After cutting, submerge the root in a cold water bath to soak for fifteen minutes. The soaking water may be used internally or externally. Burdock is fresh when it is firm and its skin is unwrinkled and taut; stored in the refrigerator wrapped in plastic, it will keep for two weeks or so. Available in some supermarkets, Japanese/Oriental markets, Korean greengrocers.

Bush Warbler Droppings : Uguisu No Fun : Sylvidae Species. Dried powdered droppings.

Cabbage/Chinese Cabbage : Kyabetsu/Hakusai : Pe Tsai : Brassica Oleracea/Brassica Campestris. Leaves. Both round-headed cabbage and Chinese cabbage, which is cylindrical, white to very pale green in color, and sweeter-tasting than the former, are used. Available at supermarkets, Oriental markets, and Korean greengrocers.

Camellia Oil : Tsubaki Abura : Camellia Linne Japonicus (Theaceae). The fruit kernels or nuts, oil pressed from the nuts. Available at some Japanese markets and at herb stores.

Carrot : Ninjin : Daucus Carota. Roots, greens. Widely available.

Castor Oil : Himashiyu : Ricinus Communis L. (Euphorbiaceae). Seeds and oil from seeds. Available at drugstores as oil, at Chinese medicine stores as seeds.

Celery : Serori/Orandamitsuba : Apium Graveolens. Greens, stems. Widely available.

Cherry Tree : Sakura : Prunus Nipponica. Bark, blossoms of the flowering cherry. The bark is available at herb stores.

Chinese Plum : Sumomo : Yu Li Ren : Prunus Japonica, P. Chinensis (Rosaceae). Fruit kernels and oil from the fruit kernels. Kernels are available from Chinese medicine stores.

Chinese Quince : Karin : Mu Gua : Chaeomeles Sinensis Koeh (Rosaceae). Fruits. Available at Chinese medicine stores.

Chlorella : Kurorera : Chlorella. Microscopic green algae, powdered. Available in natural foods stores.

Chrysanthemum : Shungiku : Ju Hua : Chrysanthemum Species (Compositae). The edible greens and yellow blossoms. Available in spring at Japanese stores and some supermarkets.

Citron : Yuzu : Citrus Medica (Rutaceae). Fruits, fruit rinds. Actually a relative of the citron, or cédrat, the *yuzu* is a yellow, rough-skinned citrus fruit about the size of a tangerine and shaped like a slightly squashed sphere. Available fresh in season in Japanese markets or as dried rind at Chinese medicine stores.

Clove : Chouji : Ding Xiang : Syzygium Aromaticum (Myrtaceae). Dried floral buds. Available at supermarkets, herb stores, and Chinese medicine stores.

Cucumber : Kyuri : Cucumis Sativus. Vegetable flesh, juice. The Japanese cucumber is smaller, has immature vestigial seeds, a thinner skin, and is crunchier than the American cucumber. The youngest and smallest of the U.S. type may substitute. Available in supermarkets and Japanese markets.

Daikon : Daikon : Raphanus Sativus L. (Crucifereae). Roots, seeds, leaves. The giant daikon radish is a white root that is generally over a foot long, weighs 4 to 5 pounds/2 kilos, and resembles the robust leg of a young girl in shape. When choosing daikon, look for firm, tight skin and a crisp, translucent white color. The white icicle radish or the largest of American white radishes may substitute. The daikon may be stored for two weeks in the refrigerator wrapped tightly in plastic, and should be grated or cut only moments before use. Dried daikon, *kiriboshi daikon*, may be stored sealed in a cool, dry location, to be soaked in tepid water for sixty minutes prior to use. Available at Japanese/Oriental markets, Korean greengrocers, natural foods stores, and Chinese medicine stores.

Dandelion : Tanpopo : Pu Gong Ying : Taraxacum Officinale Weber (Compositae). Rhizomes, roots, leaves, stem sap. Available at herb stores, Chinese medicine stores, or fresh from the garden.

Devil's Tongue Root : Konnyaku : Amorphalus Konjac. The processed roots, sold as a solid gel. Dense, dark brown, milky gray to translucent gray-white in color, *konnyaku* may appear as square cakes, balls, or noodlelike filaments. It is sold refrigerated and sitting in tubs of water, like tofu. It will keep for two weeks in the refrigerator, sitting in water that should be changed daily. To use, parboil or rinse briefly in hot water, then immerse in cold water. Tear into rough chunks. (The facial sponge described in the section on face washes may be made by using one such chunk.) Available at Japanese markets and at some natural foods stores.

Egg : Tamago. Egg whites, egg yolks. In the Japanese tradition, not only chicken eggs but quail eggs, *uzura no tamago,* are used. Quail eggs are about 1 inch/2½ cm in size, and are speckled brown and gray. They will keep for two weeks refrigerated. Quail eggs are available in some Japanese markets; chicken eggs are widely available.

Eggplant : Nasu : Solanum Melongena, S. Esculentum. Vegetable flesh, calyxes. The Japanese eggplant is about a quarter the size of the American one, is sweeter and richer in flavor, and is less grainy and less watery. The smallest American or Mediterranean eggplants may substitute. Available at some Oriental markets.

Fennel : Uikyou : Hui Xiang : Foeniculum Vulgare Mill (Umbelliferae). Fruits, seeds, leaves, stems. Available at herb stores, Chinese medicine stores, and from gardens.

Field Horsetail : Sugina : Equisetum Arvense (Equisetaceae). Stems. Available growing wild in the early spring and into summer, or at herb stores or Chinese medicine stores.

Fig : Ichijiku : Ficus Carica. Leaves, stem sap. Available in gardens and orchards.

Fish and Seafoods : Sakana; Bonito : Katsuo; Carp : Koi; Clam : Asara; Eel : Unagi; Mackerel : Saba; Oyster : Kaki; Roe : Sakana No Hararago; Sardine : Iwashi; Sea Cucumber : Namako; Sea Urchin : Uni; Shrimp : Ebi. Flesh, bones of some. Although bonito and sardines will be available in dried form at Japanese/Oriental markets, fresh fish and seafoods should be obtained in season from a fishmonger's. In cities with large Oriental communities, most of the sea creatures listed will be available.

Fruits : Kudamono. See individual listings.

Garlic : Ninniku : Allium Sativum (Liliaceae). Bulbs. Japanese garlic is milder and larger than American garlic, which may be used in its place. Available in supermarkets.

Ginger : Shoga : Gan Jiang : Zingiber Officinale Rosc (Zingiberaceae). Rhizomes. Ginger is fresh when the skin is firm and tight. Pare the thin skin only moments before use. To store, ginger may be tightly wrapped in plastic and refrigerated, kept in moist sand, or frozen. Available at supermarkets. Available in dried form at Chinese medicine stores.

Ginseng : Chousen : Ren Shen : Panax Ginseng (Araliaceae). Roots. Available at herb stores, natural foods stores, and Chinese medicine stores.

Grape : Budo : Vitus Species. Widely available.

Green Leaves : Happa.

Green Pepper : Piman : Capsicum Anuum. Vegetable flesh. The Japanese pepper is smaller, thinner-skinned, and more delicate in flavor than the American pepper, which may substitute for it. Available in supermarkets.

Honey : Hachimitsu : Feng Mi : Apis Mellifera (Apidae). Available in supermarkets, natural foods stores, and from bees.

Japanese Cypress : Hinoki : Chamaecyparis Obtusa. Aromatic wood. Available as timber from some lumberyards.

Japanese Honeysuckle : Suikazura : Jin Yin Hua : Lonicera Japonica Thunb (Caprifoliaceae). Whole plant. Japanese honeysuckle is available in gardens or at Chinese medicine stores.

Kabocha/Hokkaido Pumpkin : Kabocha : Cucurbita Moschata (Cucurbitaceae). Vegetable flesh, seeds. The *kabocha* is a green-skinned winter squash with bright, orange-yellow flesh, about 4 inches/10 cm high and about 6 inches/15 cm in diameter. It is sometimes referred to in the U.S. as Hokkaido pumpkin and sometimes as kabocha. It ripens in the autumn, and may be found in Japanese/Oriental markets at that time.

Kuzu : Kuzu : Ge Gan : Pueraria Thunbergiana Benth (Leguminosae). Processed powdered roots. This is the kudsu vine that has invaded areas of the American south and northeast. The powder of kuzu is often mistakenly identified as arrowroot. They are not the same and arrowroot should not be substituted for *kuzu*. Store well sealed in a dry location. Available at Japanese/Oriental markets and Chinese medicine stores.

Lemon : Remon : Citrus Limon. Fruits, rinds. Available at supermarkets.

Lettuce : Retasu/Chisa : Lactuca Sativa. Leaves. Widely available.

Licorice Root : Kanzou : Gan Cao : Glycyrrhiza Uralensis Fisch. G. Glabra (Leguminosae). Roots. Available at herb stores and Chinese medicine stores.

Loofah : Hechima : Si Gua Luo : Luffa Cylindrica Roem., L. Aegyptiaca (Cucurbitaceae). Fruit fibers, vine sap. Available as dried washing sponge at natural foods stores, specialty shops, and bath goods shops. The vine sap may be collected from a live plant.

Lotus : Renkon : He Ye : Nelumbo Nucifera (Nymphaeaceae). Whole plant, especially the roots. A picturesque vegetable, lotus root comes in links, each about 5 inches/13 cm long and 2½ inches/6½ cm in diameter. When fresh, the color is ivory white and firm. The root may be stored like potatoes, but once cut, the remaining portion should be used within a day or two. To prepare, pare the skin with a potato peeler, slice, and immerse in vinegared or salted cold water for thirty minutes. It must be used shortly thereafter. Dried lotus root must be soaked for two hours and drained before use. Lotus root is available fresh in fall and winter at Japanese/Oriental markets.

Melon : Meron/Makuwauri : Cucurbitaceae Family. Flesh, seeds. While certain Japanese melons are not available in the United States, in general the cantaloupe, honeydew, and Persian melons may be used instead. Available in supermarkets.

Millet : Kibi : Panicum Miliaceum. Grains. Millet is available at natural foods stores and is sold as birdseed in pet shops.

Mountain Yam/Chinese Yam : Jinenjo/Yamaimo/Nagaimo : Shan Yao : Dioscorea Japonica Thunb., D. Opposita (Dioscoreaceae). Tubers. The mountain yam is light brown and hairy-skinned, an irregularly shaped and exceedingly long root that can reach a yard/meter in length. To store, wrap in plastic and refrigerate for up to two weeks. Available growing wild in parts of America, and in Japanese markets and some natural foods stores.

Mugwort : Yomogi : Ai Ye : Artemisia Vulgaris L. (Compositae). Leaves. Mugwort is available growing wild, in herb stores, and in Chinese medicine stores.

Mustard : Karashi : Brassica Nigra. Seeds. Japanese mustard is sold powdered or as a paste, and is very hot. English or Chinese mustard may substitute. Available at Japanese/Oriental markets.

Olive Oil : Oriibu Oiru : Olea Europaea. Oil from the fruits. Only the purest extra virgin olive oil should be used. In natural foods stores, olive oil by Haines, Carothers, or Walnut Acres are good quality.

Onion : Tamanegi : Allium Cepa. Bulbs. Widely available.

Orange : Orenji : Zhi Shi : Citrus Family. Fruits—ripe and unripe—and rinds. Available at greengrocers.

Peach : Momo : Tao Ren : Prunus Persica Batsch (Rosaceae). Fruits, leaves, fruit kernels. The fruit kernel is poisonous in large doses. The fruits are available at markets, while the leaves are available from trees, and the kernel form is available at Chinese medicine stores.

Pear : Nashi : Pyrus Communis. Fruits. Widely available.

Pearl : Shinju; Pearl Oyster Shell : Kaki No Kai : Mu Li : Ostrea Rivularis (Ostreidae). Powdered pearls, powdered shells. Available in powdered form at Chinese medicine stores.

Pearl Barley/Job's Tears : Hatomugi : Yi Yi Ren : Coix Lacrymae Jobi L. (Graminae). Seeds. Available at natural foods stores as grain and flour, and at Chinese medicine stores.

Perilla : Shiso : Zi Su : Perilla Frutescens Britt (Labiatae). Leaves, seeds, stems. When buying the fresh leaf, make sure it is not wilted. Available growing wild, or in Japanese markets in both green and red forms. Available at Chinese medicine stores.

Persimmon/Japanese Persimmon : Kaki : Shi Di : Diospyros Kaki (Ebenaceae). Fruits, calyxes, leaves. The Japanese persimmon exists in a squarish shape and an elongated plumlike one. Persimmons are picked when firm rather than soft. The astringent skin must be removed prior to use. In Japan, persimmon leaf tea is sold as *kaki no hacha*. Available from trees (American persimmons may substitute), occasionally in autumn at Japanese/Oriental markets, or at Chinese medicine stores.

Pine : Matsu : Pinus Family. Needles, resin. Available from trees.

Plum ("Ume") Products

Plum: Ume : Prunus Mume Sieb. Et Zucc (Rosaceae). Unripe fruits, fruit kernels, blossoms. This is actually a type of apricot, though popularly referred to in English as a plum. *Ume*, which resemble apricots in shape and size, fall from the tree when they are unripe, hard, bright green and sour. (If weather conditions allow the fruits to remain on the tree to ripen, they become yellow-apricot in color, soft and sweet.) Unripe *ume* are available fresh in Japanese markets in June, and the blossoms and fruits are available from trees.

Pickled Plum : Umeboshi. A sour, red, wrinkled ball made by steeping unripe *ume* in brine and red perilla. Available at Japanese markets and natural foods stores.

Plum Extract : Bainikuekisu. A sour concentrate made by cooking down the flesh of unripe *ume*. Available at Japanese markets, natural foods stores.

Plum Vinegar : Umesu. The brine obtained after steeping ume to make *umeboshi*. Available at Japanese markets.

Plum Liquor : Umeshu. A sweet alcoholic beverage made by steeping unripe *ume* in *shochu* with rock sugar. Ingredients available at Japanese markets.

Potato : Jagaimo : Solanum Tuberosum : Tubers. Though there are slight differences between the most commonly used Japanese potatoes and the American potato varieties, they may be considered interchangeable. Available at markets.

Rice And Rice Products

Rice : Kome : Oryza Sativa L. (Graminae). Grains, germinated seeds, bran. Whole-grain rice is *genmai* in Japanese. Available at natural foods stores.

Rice Bran : Komenuka. Rice bran sold for pickling often contains additives—red peppers, sweet wine, salt—and so is not appropriate for other uses. Pure fresh rice bran is available from grain stores and natural foods stores.

Rice Flour : Joshinko/Mochiko/Shiratamako. Joshinko is ground from uncooked white rice. *Mochiko* is ground from dried cooked glutinous rice (*mochigome*). *Shiratamako* is ground from uncooked glutinous rice. Brown rice flour is the ground whole grain. Rice flour is available at Japanese/Oriental markets and natural foods stores.

Rice Vinegar : Komezu. Vinegar made from rice, white or brown. Available at Japanese markets and natural foods stores.

Rice Wine : Sake. A dry alcoholic beverage containing 15 to 17 percent alcohol, not a wine but often classified as such. *Sake* should be stored in a cool, dark location. A *sake* made from brown rice without additives is made in the United States by Kimoto Brewing Company, Berthoud, Colorado. Ordinary *sake* is available at liquor stores and Japanese markets.

Rose : Bara : Rosa Species (Rosaceae). Flowers. Available from gardens, at herb stores and Chinese medicine stores.

Safflower : Benibana : Hong Hua : Carthamus Tinctorius L. (Compositae). Flowers, seeds, oil pressed from the seeds. The flowers are available in gardens, at herb stores and Chinese medicine stores. High-quality oil is available at natural foods stores.

Saffron : Safuran: Crocus Sativas. Stamens. Available at gourmet food stores and herb stores.

Salt : Shio : Sodium Chloride. Sea Salt is the preferred variety. Available at gourmet foods stores and natural foods stores.

Sandalwood : Byakudan : Santalum Album L. (Santalaceae). Aromatic wood. Available at herb stores and Chinese medicine stores.

Sea Plants

Sea Plants Kaiso. Because many sea plants sold in the United States are of Japanese origin or used in Japanese cooking, these are often labeled with the Anglicized Japanese name, thus the Japanese name is likely to be most familiar to readers. The following plants are therefore classified according to their most commonly known names, whether English or Japanese.

Arame : Eisenia Bicyclis, E. Arborea. Delicate filaments of shredded *arame* leaf. Available at Japanese markets and natural foods stores.

Dulse : Palmaria Palmata. Leaves, purplish-red in color. Available at natural foods stores.

Funori : Gloiopeltis Furcata. Purplish-red leaves, stems, and pods. Available at natural foods stores.

Hijiki : Hizikia Fusiformis. Whole plant. Tubular, narrow, curly black strands. Available at Japanese markets and natural foods stores.

Irish Moss : Chondrus Crispus. Whole plant. Available at natural foods stores.

Kelp : Kombu : Laminaria Japonica Aresch (Laminariaceae). Whole plant. Also known as "sea tangle," *kombu* is olive brown to deep green in color, with very wide, long leaves. Wipe with a damp cloth prior to use. Available at Japanese markets and natural foods stores.

Laver : Nori : Porphyra Tenera. Whole plant. Sold in green-black sheets or as leaves. Available at Japanese markets, natural foods stores. The green *nori* flakes sold as *aonori* are from the plant *porphyra enteromorpha*.

Tengusa : Gelidium Amansii. Whole plant. Used in making gelatin, this plant is translucent white or pinkish-red, sold in long strips. Available at Japanese markets and natural foods stores.

Wakame : Undaria Pinnatifida. Whole plant. Long bright green leaves. American *alaria*, *alaria marginata* may substitute. Available at Japanese markets and natural foods stores.

Note: All sea plants must be stored in a cool, dark, dry location.

Seashells : Kai. Aromatic conch and spiral shells, powdered. Available at Chinese medicine stores.

Sesame : Goma : Sesamum Indicum L. (Pedaliaceae). Seeds, oil pressed from the seeds. Sesame seeds exist in black—*kurogoma*—and white varieties. Both types are commonly roasted slightly before use. Sesame oil, *goma abura*, is available in three forms: light roasted, dark roasted, and "hot" roasted, which contains red pepper and is usually Chinese. Sesame seeds should be stored in a cool, dark location. Oils produced by Ohsawa, Arrowhead Mills, Erewhon, and Haines are high quality. Available at Japanese markets, gourmet foods stores, natural foods stores.

Sharks's Liver Oil : Same No Kimo No Yu. Shark's liver oil, also referred to as *squalene*, may be available at some natural foods stores.

Shiitake Mushrooms : Shiitake : Lentinus Edodes, Cortinellis Shiitake. Mushrooms. Sometimes marketed in America as "black forest shiitake," the mushrooms are large, with caps of about 2 inches/5 cm in diameter, a velvety-brown on top and with creamy white undersides. When choosing fresh shiitake, look for no discoloration of the white underside of the cap, and the mushroom should not seem thin, sagging, or shriveled. Dried mushrooms should have caps that turn under. Fresh mushrooms will last for a few days refrigerated, but are best used immediately. Dried mushrooms will last indefinitely if stored well sealed in a cool, dry location. They may be soaked in water overnight; save soaking water for later use. Shiitake mushrooms are available at supermarkets, Japanese/Oriental markets, and natural foods stores.

Shochu. Also known as "white liquor," *shochu* is a distilled spirit containing 20 to 45 percent alcohol. It is tasteless and odorless. Vodka may substitute for it in the recipes in this book. Available at some liquor stores and at Japanese markets.

Soybeans and Soybean Products

Soybean : Daizu : Glycine Max, G. Soja. Seeds. Soybeans are small, round yellowish beans when dried; when fresh, they are often sold in their pods, which are bright green like the soft legumes inside. Available at supermarkets, Japanese/ Oriental markets, and natural foods stores.

Bean Curd : Tofu. The square white cakes of bean curd sold in American stores immersed in water will last for about five days if refrigerated immersed in water which is changed daily. Available at supermarkets, Japanese/Oriental markets, and Korean greengrocers.

Bean Sprouts : Moyashi. The familiar bean sprout is widely available at supermarkets, Japanese/Oriental markets, and natural foods stores.

Miso. Fermented soybean paste, miso exists in a range of colors and flavors, with white, yellow, red, and dark brown varieties each having its own distinct richness and strength. Miso will keep for up to a year in the refrigerator. Available at Japanese markets and natural foods stores.

Natto. A fermented soybean product, cheesy-smelling and gooey. Fresh, *natto* will last for a week in the refrigerator. Frozen *natto* may be kept indefinitely; thaw immediately prior to use. Available in Japanese markets and natural foods stores.

Okara. A crumbly, moist whitish substance that is the pulp left over from making tofu. It is available fresh wherever tofu is produced. *Okara* must be refrigerated. Available at Japanese markets or at a tofu-producer's.

Soy Oil : Daizu Abura. Oil made from the soybean. Available at supermarkets and natural foods stores.

215

Soybean Flour : Kinako. Flour made from roasted and ground soybeans. *Kinako* is available at Japanese markets and natural foods stores.

Soybean Vinegar : Sudaizu. Vinegar containing whole soybeans. Available at Japanese markets.

Soy Sauce : Shoyu. Soy sauce is widely available, but the best types are made by natural methods, such as those by Mitoku or Ohsawa, available at natural foods stores.

Spinach : Horenso : Spinacia Oleracea. Leaves. Japanese spinach is similar to American spinach; they may be used interchangeably. Available at supermarkets and Korean greengrocers.

Strawberry : Ichigo : Frageria Vesca. Fruits. Available at markets and in gardens.

Sweet Flag : Shobu : A Species of Iris (Iridaceae). Flowers, leaves, stems, roots. Purple to white blossoms and sharp-pointed, flat leaves that resemble swords. Available in gardens.

Tangerine : Mikan : Chen Pi : Citrusreticulata (Rutaceae). Fruits, fruit rinds, seeds, leaves. The dried, ground peel is known as *chinpi* in Japanese. The Japanese tangerine or mandarin orange is a winter fruit, small, a squashed sphere in shape, with a loose skin and sweet flavor. Both fruit and rind are vivid orange in color. Available fresh at Korean greengrocers, supermarkets, and Japanese/Oriental markets. The dried peel is available at Chinese medicine stores.

Taro : Satoimo : Colocasia Esculenta. Tubers. Taro, also known as yams, are small, with dark brown skins which must be scraped or pared prior to use. Available fresh during the winter at Japanese/Oriental markets.

Tea

Tea : Cha : Thea Sinensis L. (Theaceae). Leaves, stems, twigs. All of the teas come from the same plant, with the difference in color, aroma, taste, and caffeine content being due to differences in processing as well as the portion of the plant employed. In Japan, varieties of green tea are drunk most commonly, with Chinese black teas popular as well. All teas are available in loose leaf form at Japanese/Oriental markets, with some available at natural foods stores or gourmet foods stores.

Black Teas : Oolong and Po Lei. Both are Chinese teas.

Green Teas : Ocha. The many grades and varieties fall into the following categories:

Gyokuro. Made from the highest, earliest tender leaves, this is the finest of the green teas.

Matcha. This powdered *gyokuro*, used in the tea ceremony.

Sencha. Made from leaves lower on the plant, this is medium-grade green tea.

Bancha. Made from the lowest leaves and small twigs, this is the lowest grade green tea with the least amount of caffeine.

Hojicha. Roasted *bancha* tea.

Genmai-Cha. Bancha mixed with roasted puffed brown rice kernels.

Kukicha. Not a true green tea, this is made from the final cutting of the tea plant, using twigs and stems only. It is boiled, not steeped.

   Note: All teas must be stored well sealed in cool, dry locations.

Tomato : Tomato : Lycopersicum Esculentum. Vegetable flesh. available at greengrocers.

Turnip: Kabu : Brassica Rapa. Roots, greens. The Japanese turnip is pure white and 2 inches/5 cm or so in diameter. American turnips may substitute. Available at supermarkets.

Walnut : Kurumi : Juglans Nigra, J. Mandshurica (Juglandiaceae). Hulls, kernels, leaves. Walnuts and walnut oil are available in supermarkets.

Wasabi : Wasabi : Wasabia Japonica. Roots. Sold fresh, the *wasabi* root is brown outside, green inside, about 4 inches/10 cm in length, and about 1 inch/2½ cm in width at the widest point. It must be stored in water and refrigerated. Pare the skin prior to use. *Wasabi* is also available as a paste in tubes or as a powder. The paste must be refrigerated. Available at Japanese markets and natural foods stores.

Watermelon : Suika : Citrullus Vulgaris Schrad (Cucurbitaceae). Flesh, rinds, seeds. Rind and seeds are available at Chinese medicine stores; whole fruits are available at supermarkets.

Wheat : Komugi : Xiao Mai : Triticum Vulgare, T. Aestivum (Graminae). Grains, bran. Available at natural foods stores and Chinese medicine stores.

BOOKS OF INTEREST

Japanese Foods and Cooking

Cooking With Japanese Foods: A Guide to the Traditional Natural Foods of Japan by Jan and John Belleme, East-West Health Books, Brookline, MA, 1986

Japanese Home Style Cooking ed. Mihoko Hoshino, Better Home Publishing House, Tokyo, 1986

Japanese Cooking for Health and Fitness by Kiyoko Konshi, Gakken, Tokyo, 1983

A First Book of Japanese Cooking by Yamaoka Masako, Kodansha International, Tokyo, 1984

Colette's Japanese Cuisine by Colette Rossant, Kodansha International, Tokyo, 1985

Japanese Cooking: A Simple Art by Shizuo Tsuji, Kodansha International, Tokyo, 1980

Hyakumi Saisai: Innovative Vegetable Cuisine From Japan by Fukiko Yokoyama, Libroport, Tokyo, 1990

The Japanese Bath

Furo: The Japanese Bath by Peter Grilli and Dana Levy, Kodansha International, Tokyo, 1985

A Guide to Japanese Hot Springs by Anne Hotta with Yoko Ishiguro, Kodansha International, Tokyo, 1986

Traditions of Discipline and Practice

Judo: The Gentle Way by Alan Fromm and Nicholas Soames, Arkana, London, 1988

T'ai Chi Chuan and Meditation by Da Liu, Arkana, London, 1988

Cha-No-Yu: The Japanese Tea Ceremony by A. L. Sadler, Tuttle, Tokyo, 1962

Chado: The Japanese Way of Tea by Soshitsu Sen, Weatherhill, Tokyo, 1979

The Tea Ceremony by Tanaka Sen'o, Kodansha International, Tokyo, 1983

Chanoyu: The Urasenke Tradition of Tea ed. Soshitsu Sen XV, Weatherhill, Tokyo, 1988

Zen and the Art of Calligraphy by Omori Sogen and Terayama Katsujo, Arkana, London, 1988

❀

Traditional Healing: Tsubo and Herbs

Natural Healers' Acupressure Handbook Volume I: *Basic G-Jo*; Volume II: *Advanced G-Jo* by Michael Blate, Arkana, London, 1988

Shiatzu: Japanese Finger Pressure for Energy, Sexual Vitality, and Relief from Tension and Pain
by Yukiko Irwin with James Wagenvoord, Arkana, London, 1991

Chinese Herbs by John D. Keys, Tuttle, Tokyo, 1976

Chinese Massage Therapy: A Handbook of Therapeutic Massage Compiled at the Anhui Medical School, Hospital, China Translated by Hor Ming Lee and Gregory Whincup, Arkana, London, 1988

The Complete Book of Shiatsu Therapy by Toru Namikoshi, Japan Publications, Tokyo, 1981

Chinese Herbal Medicine by Daniel P. Reid, Shambhala, Boston, 1987

Massage: The Oriental Methods by Katsusuke Serizawa, M.D., Japan Publications, Tokyo, 1972

Tsubo: Vital Points for Oriental Therapy by Katsusuke Serizawa, M.D., Japan Publications, Tokyo, 1976

Effective Tsubo Therapy by Katsusuke Serizawa, M.D., Japan Publications, Tokyo, 1984

The Layman's Guide to Acupuncture by Manaka Yoshio, M.D., and Ian A. Urquhart, Ph.D., Weatherhill, Tokyo, 1972

Beauty of the Spirit

Zen Seeds: Reflections of a Female Priest by Shundo Aoyama, translated by Patricia Daien Bennage, Kosei, Tokyo, 1990

Weavers of Wisdom: Women Mystics of the Twentieth Century by Anne Bancroft, Arkana, London, 1989

Woman Awake: A Celebration of Women's Wisdom by Christina Feldman, Arkana, London, 1989

Even in Summer the Ice Doesn't Melt by David K. Reynolds, Ph.D., Quill, William Morrow, New York, 1986

Tea Life, Tea Mind by Soshitsu Sen XV, Weatherhill, Tokyo, 1979

A Gathering of Spirit: Women Teaching in American Buddhism ed. Ellen Sidor, Primary Point Press, Rhode Island, 1987

REFERENCES

Basho, Matsuo. *On Love and Barley: Haiku of Basho.* Translated by Lucien Stryk. London: Penguin, 1988.

Basho, Matsuo. *A Haiku Journey: Basho's Narrow Road to a Far Province.* Translated by D.G. Britton. Tokyo: Kodansha International, 1980.

Belleme, Jan and John. *Cooking With Japanese Foods: A Guide to the Traditional Natural Foods of Japan.* Brookline, Mass.: East-West Health Books, 1986.

Bremness, Lesley. *Pocket Encyclopedia of Herbs.* London: Dorling Kindersley, 1990.

Chikamatsu, Monzaemon. *Koushoku Ichidai Onna.* Excerpted in *Keshoshi Bunken Shiryo Nenpyo.* Tokyo: Pola Bunka Kenkyujo, 1979. NKBT*

Chotto Obaachan Oshiete. Edited by Mainichi Shimbun, Shakai-bu. Tokyo: Bunka Shuppan Kyoku, 1986.

Dalby, Liza. *Geisha.* New York: Vintage Books, 1985.

Dazai, Osamu. "Memories." *A Late Chrysanthemum.* Translated by Lane Dunlop. Tokyo: Charles E. Tuttle, 1988.

Dazai, Osamu. *The Setting Sun.* Translated by Donald Keene. Tokyo: Charles E. Tuttle, 1989.

Dyer, Sarah. *A Pocket Book on Herbs.* London: Octopus Books, 1982.

Ehon Edomurasaki. Excerpted in *Keshoshi Bunken Shiryo Nenpyo.* Tokyo: Pola Bunka Kenkyujo, 1979.

Ejima, Kiseki. *Keisei Kintanki.* Excerpted in *Keshoshi Bunken Shiryo Nenpyo.* Tokyo: Pola Bunka Kenkyujo, 1979. NKBT*

Ekiguchi, Kunio and Ruth McCreery. *A Japanese Touch for the Seasons.* Tokyo: Kodansha International, 1989.

Fujiwara, Tokihira, Tadahira, et al. *Engishiki.* Excerpted in *Keshoshi Bunken Shiryo Nenpyo.* Tokyo: Pola Bunka Kenkyujo, 1979.

Haikara-Modan Keshoshi. Edited by Pola Bunka Kenkyujo. Tokyo: Pola Bunka Kenkyujo, 1986.

Hayashi, Fumiko. "A Late Chrysanthemum." *A Late Chrysanthemum,* Translated by Lane Dunlop. Tokyo: Charles E. Tuttle, 1988.

Hearn, Lafcadio. *A Japanese Miscellany.* Tokyo: Charles E. Tuttle, 1982.

Hearn, Lafcadio. *Glimpses of Unfamiliar Japan.* Tokyo: Charles E. Tuttle, 1984.

Hearn, Lafcadio. *Shadowings.* Tokyo: Charles E. Tuttle, 1971.

Hiratsuka, Raicho. *Bluestocking,* Vol. 1, No. 1. Tokyo: Seito-Sha, 1911.

Hiroidama Shin Chienoumi. Excerpted in *Keshoshi Bunken Shiryo Nenpyo.* Tokyo: Pola Bunka Kenkyujo, 1979.

Hotta, Anne and Yoko Ishiguro. *A Guide to Japanese Hot Springs.* Tokyo: Kodansha International, 1986.

Ikeda, Daisaku. *Glass Children.* Tokyo: Kodansha International, 1983.

Inishie no Roman. Edited by Benibana Shiryokan. Kahokucho: Kahokucho Kyoiku Iinkai, 1989.

Isoho Monogatari. Excerpted in *Keshoshi Bunken Shiryo Nenpyo.* Tokyo: Pola Bunka Kenkyujo, 1979. NKBT*

Isoda, Doji. *Chikusai.* Excerpted in *Keshoshi Bunken Shiryo Nenpyo.* Tokyo: Pola Bunka Kenkyujo, 1979. NKBT*

Ishikawa, Takuboku. *Romaji Diary and Sad Toys.* Translated by Sanford Goldstein and Seishi Shinoda. Tokyo: Charles E. Tuttle, 1985.

James, Grace. *Green Willow and Other Japanese Fairy Tales.* New York: Avenel Books, 1987.

Kawabata, Yasunari. *Beauty and Sadness.* Translated by Howard Hibbett. London: Penguin, 1979.

Kawabata, Yasunari. *Snow Country.* Translated by Edward G. Seidensticker. Tokyo: Charles E. Tuttle, 1983.

Kazantzakis, Nikos. *Japan China*. Berkeley: Creative Arts Books Company, 1982.

Kenko. *Essays in Idleness: The Tsurezuregusa of Kenko*. Translated by Donald Keene. Tokyo: Charles E. Tuttle, 1989.

Kenton, Leslie. *The Joy of Beauty*. London: Arrow Books, 1989.

Keys, John D. *Chinese Herbs*. Tokyo: Charles E. Tuttle, 1990.

Kou to Koudou. Edited by Koudou Bunka Kenkyukai. Tokyo: Yuuzankaku Shuppan, 1989.

Krouse, Carolyn R. *A Guide to Food Buying in Japan*. Tokyo: Charles E. Tuttle, 1986.

Kuahausu Jigyo Kaihatsu Manyuaru. Edited by Nihon Kenko Kaihatsu Zaidan. Tokyo: Nihon Kenko Kaihatsu Zaidan. 1987.

Matsue, Shigeyori. *Kefukigusa*. Excerpted in *Keshoshi Bunken Shiryo Nenpyo*. Tokyo: Pola Bunka Kenkyujo, 1979. IB*

Mayhew, Lenore, translator. *Monkey's Raincoat*. Tokyo: Charles E. Tuttle, 1985.

Mizushima, Uraya. *Kewai Mayutsukuri Kuden*. Excerpted in *Keshoshi Bunken Shiryo Nenpyo*. Tokyo: Pola Bunka Kenkyujo, 1979.

Morishita, Keichi. *Yakukoshoku*. Tokyo: Hakuju-Sha, 1986.

Morris, Ivan. *The World of the Shining Prince*. London: Peregrine Books, 1979.

Murasaki, Shikibu. *The Tale of Genji*. Translated by Arthur Waley. Tokyo: Charles E. Tuttle, 1990.

Murasawa, Hiroto and Norio Tsuda, editors. *Keshoshi Bunken Shiryo Nenpyo*. Tokyo: Pola Bunka Kenkyujo, 1979.

Murata, Takako, Norio Tsuda, Hiromi Yamamura, and Eri Tamaru, editors. *Nihon no Kesho*. Tokyo: Pola Bunka Kenkyujo, 1989.

Namiki, Shouzou and Kouzou Asano. *Yougan Bienkou*. Excerpted in *Keshoshi Bunken Shiryo Nenpyo*. Tokyo: Pola Bunka Kenkyujo, 1979.

Namikoshi, Toru. *The Complete Book of Shiatsu Therapy*. Tokyo: Japan Publications, 1981.

Okakura, Kakuzo. *The Book of Tea*. Tokyo: Charles E. Tuttle, 1960.

Okuda, Shouhaken, editor. *Onna Youkin Mouzui*. Tokyo: Kaseigaku Bunkenshusei. Excerpted in *Keshoshi Bunken Shiryo Nenpyo*. Tokyo: Pola Bunka Kenkyujo, 1979.

Onna Chouhouki. Excerpted in *Keshoshi Bunken Shiryo Nenpyo*. Tokyo: Pola Bunka Kenkyujo, 1979. NDL*

Onna Kagami Hidensho. Excerpted in *Heshoshi Bunken Shiryo Nenpyo*. Tokyo: Pola Bunka Kenkyujo, 1979. NDL*

Otomo, Yakamochi et al, editors. *Manyoshu*. Excerpted in *Keshoshi Bunken Shiryo Nenpyo*. Tokyo: Pola Bunka Kenkyujo, 1979. NKBT*

Reid, Daniel P. *Chinese Herbal Medicine*. Boston: Shambhala, 1987.

Reynolds, David K. *Even in Summer the Ice Doesn't Melt*. New York: Quill, 1986.

Rose, Jeanne. *Jeanee Rose's Herbal Body Book*. New York: Perigree, 1982.

Sawa, Yuki and Edith M. Shiffert. *Haiku Master Buson*. San Francisco: Heian International, 1978.

Sayama, Hanshichimaru. *Miyako Fuuzoku Keshouden*. Excerpted in *Keshoshi Bunken Shiryo Nenpyo*. Tokyo: Pola Bunka Kenkyujo, 1979.

Serizawa, Katsusuke M.D. *Effective Tsubo Therapy*. Tokyo: Japan Publications, 1984.

Serizawa, Katsusuke M.D. *Massage: The Oriental Methods*. Tokyo: Japan Publications, 1972.

Serizawa, Katsusuke M.D. *Tsubo: Vital Points for Oriental Therapy*. Tokyo: Japan Publications, 1976.

Shigematsu, Soiku. *A Zen Harvest: Japanese Folk Zen Sayings*. San Francisco: North Point Press, 1988.

Shonagon, Sei. *The Pillow Book of Sei Shonagon*. Translated by Ivan Morris. London: Penguin, 1984.

Sou, Keisei, editor. *Tenkou Kaibutsu*. Tokyo: Touyou Bunko Heibonsha. Excerpted in *Keshoshi Bunken Shiryo Nenpyo*, 1979.

Takahashi, Yumiko. *Shimi, Shiwa o Totte, Kireini Wakagaeru*. Tokyo: Shufonotomo-Sha, 1984.

Tamenaga, Shunsui. *Shunshoku Tatsumino Sono*. Excerpted in *Keshoshi Bunken Shiryo Nenpyo*. Tokyo: Pola Bunka Kenkyujo, 1979. NKBT*

Tanizaki, Junichiro. *In Praise of Shadows*. Translated by Thomas J. Harper and Edward G. Seidensticker. Tokyo: Charles E. Tuttle, 1990.

Tanizaki, Junichiro. "The Tattooer." *Seven Japanese Tales by Junichiro Tanizaki*. Translated by Howard Hibbett. New York: Putnam, 1981.

Taneda, Santoka. *Mountain Tasting*. Translated by John Stevens. Tokyo: Weatherhill, 1989.

Tawara, Machi. *Salad Anniversary*. Translated by Juliet Winters Carpenter. Tokyo: Kodansha International, 1989.

Terashima. Ryouan. *Wakansansaizue*. Tokyo: Nihon Zuihitsu Taisei Bekkan. Excerpted in *Keshoshi Bunken Shiryo Nenpyo*. Tokyo: Pola Bunka Kenkyujo, 1979.

Torikaebaya Monogatari. Tokyo: Kouchuu Nihon Bungaku Taikei. Excerpted in *Keshoshi Bunken Shiryo Nenpyo*, Tokyo: Pola Bunka Kenkyujo, 1979.

Tsuda, Norio and Takako Murata. *Mayu no Bunkashi (Mayu Kesho Kenkyu Hokokusho)*. Tokyo: Pola Bunka Kenkyujo, 1984.

Tsuda, Norio and Takako Murata. *Modan Keshoshi*. Tokyo: Pola Bunka Kenkyujo, 1986.

Tsuji, Shizuo. *Japanese Cooking: A Simple Art*. Tokyo: Kodansha International, 1984.

Tsutui, Shoushi. *Mukashi Kara Tsutae Rarete Iru: Shizen Butsu de Bihada Zukuri O*. Ushiyama: Biyou Bunka-Sha.

Uno, Chiyo. *Confessions of Love*. Translated by Phyllis Birnbaum. Tokyo: Charles E. Tuttle, 1990.

Watashi No Kenko. (Issues published between 1985–1990.) Tokyo: Shufunotomo-Sha.

Wyman, Donald. *Wyman's Gardening Encyclopedia*. New York: Macmillan, 1986.

Yamada, Ei. *Shizenkeshohin no Himitsu*. Tokyo: Nagaoka Shoten, 1984.

Yamada, Kyoko. *Biyo to Shokuji No Daikenkyu*. Tokyo: Sanpo-Sha, 1981.

Yosano, Akiko. *Tangled Hair (Selected Tanka From Midaregami)*. Translated by Sanford Goldstein and Seishi Shinoda. Tokyo: Charles E. Tuttle, 1987.

Yuu Kouro: Nihongami wa Kataru. Tokyo: Pola Bunka Kenkyujo, 1985.

Zouhou Hiroidama Chienoumi. Excerpted in *Keshoshi Bunken Shiryo Nenpyo*, Tokyo: Pola Bunka Kenkyujo, 1979.

*NOTE: Sources compiled in *Keshoshi Bunken Shiryo Nenpyo* were gathered by Pola researchers from a wide variety of sources. Where the information regarding the original source of the full-length work is available, I have indicated it at the end of the entry with abbreviations:

NDL: New Diet Library, Tokyo. These works are rare, sometimes existing only as handwritten manuscripts.

NKBT: *Nihon Kotenbungaku Taikei*. Tokyo: Iwanami Shoten.

IB: *Iwanami Bunko*. Tokyo: Iwanami Shoten.

ACKNOWLEDGMENTS

The Japanese way of beauty exists as folk wisdom stored in the memories of the oldest living Japanese women. It is the knowledge these women shared with me that forms the core of the book. For the information thus gathered, often in the course of a casual conversation, a chance encounter, a spontaneous reminiscence, I wish to acknowledge and thank the many beautiful Japanese grandmothers I have had the honor to meet.

In the work of literary research, translation, and verification of facts, I also received invaluable assistance from many young Japanese women. I wish to thank Megumi Abe; Masami Ito; Rikiko Matsuda; Shizuko Kanehira; Miyuki Mito; Yoshiko Ishihara; Ikuko Yamamoto; Yuka Yoshida; Sakiko Kumagai; Mariko Kaneta; Yumiko Sugai; Sachiko Kimura; Michiko Hirose; Keiko Omiya; and Makiko Kaneyama, all of whom helped me immeasurably. I wish to thank Mari Kato for her diligent assistance in tracking down obscure facts about Asian herbs, and I wish to thank Ryo Takahashi for her contribution of pharmaceutical knowledge of plants used traditionally in women's beauty. I particularly wish to recognize and thank Michiko Kohama for her faithful and untiring help in translation and research, and for her perceptive advice in a wide range of areas. I wish to thank the midwives Haru Karube and Julie Pearse for their assistance and their knowledge of female folk traditions.

The mothers and grandmothers of many of my assistants contributed a wealth of knowledge, of which often even their own daughters had been unaware. Many fathers, grandfathers, and husbands supplied the important male perspective on feminine beauty.

Setsuko Tanezawa has served as an inspiring example of harmonious inner and outer beauty; Fusako Tamiya taught me that the ritual of the tea ceremony may be made a part of real life; Tatsuro Ishii imparted his insights into ancient Shinto and shamanesses; Kim Schuefftan offered important support and enthusiasm when the book was a nascent idea.

I wish to thank Takako Murata of Pola for her generous and learned assistance; Shu Uemura for sharing his thoughts on women's beauty; Takashi Morigaki and Chieko and Steven Weiler of Yuen Cosmetics for their enthusiastic assistance. Irina and Takahisa Yokoyama offered multidimensional help; Melissa and Phiya Kushi and Michio and Aveline Kushi shared their knowledge of Japanese natural foods and the traditional lifestyle. Bill Truesdale of New Rivers Press, Tom Chapman of Emphasis, and Mac and Romi Davis of MacDavis are thanked wholeheartedly for their ongoing support of my creative endeavors. Leslie Kenton has been a generous source of inspiration. William Miller, Rebecca Gleason, and Alison Bond are to be thanked for their dedicated and patient support in helping to bring the project to fruition. I am grateful to Gail Kinn, my editor, for her remarkable work in shaping my manuscript into an object of understated Japanese beauty.

I wish to thank Linda Sugawara, Kelly Miller, Naomi and Lisa Mandeville, Yaiko Otomo, Becky Shidara, David Tate, Lucia Kellar, and Theodosia Greene, each of whom offered important help when it was most needed. I wish to thank Hiro Ota for finding me a writing room in an ancient samurai garden, supplying me with a reliable typewriter, and introducing me to the spirit of Japan.

To my international extended family—Jack and Song Sun Anderson, Joy Anderson and Don Hauser, Dolly Coonrad, Tina and Andre Firmignac, Mei Mei Anderson, Jon and Erica Anderson, Scott Anderson, Marilyn and Frank Amantia, Judi and Steven Kaplan, George and Dorothy Leigh—I offer another resounding thank you. And to Gabriel, Amber, and Bruce, thank you, thank you, and thank you again.

ADVICE FROM JAPANESE GRANDMOTHERS
ON HOW TO BE BEAUTIFUL

Protect your skin from the sun.

Drink pure water, breathe good air, live in a clean house.

As you grow older, don't envy the fresh blossoms of spring.

To have clear, smooth skin, care for it diligently by cleaning it completely, protecting it with loofah vine-water, and keeping a relaxed mind.

Good skin comes from a clean body, so make sure to eat foods that purify the body.

Eat the peels, rinds, and skins of fruits and vegetables.

Too much makeup pollutes the skin.

If your bad skin is inherited, you can change its condition by eating properly.

Sleep at least eight hours a night, and go to bed before eleven.

Be in love.

Be active. Get exercise. Enjoy your life.

Don't sit around worrying.

Control your desires. Don't always want what you can't have. This unsatisfied yearning habit makes a woman ugly.

Accept your age and the changes in your beauty.

A beautiful old woman is beautiful because her mind and spirit are wise and graceful.

At the age of forty, the mind is visible on the face.

Practice facial massage every day to prevent wrinkles, lines, and age spots, and to keep the skin fresh and supple.

If you are tired or suffering from stress, you must exercise.

Eat a wide variety of foods.

Don't complain; don't be envious; don't be irritated. Your health will deteriorate and your skin will look terrible.

If your shoulders are tense or stiff, you will have lines and wrinkles on your face. Practice massage.

Enjoy lovemaking. You will have glowing, shiny skin and a relaxed face.

Enjoy nature. Be tranquil and calm. Eat simple foods.

You can tighten your skin by massaging it: face, head, and neck.

If you breathe deeply, you'll become strong and healthy and more attractive.

Everybody gets wrinkles, but try to prevent ugly wrinkles by controlling your mind and emotions. Wrinkles are a reflection of your thoughts and feelings.

Clean skin, not makeup, is the secret of beautiful skin.

If you just cleanse, nourish, and massage your skin, it will function well and look good.